THE SPIRITUAL DENTIST

Discovering the Hidden Wisdom of Oral Health

Dr. Mitu Singhal

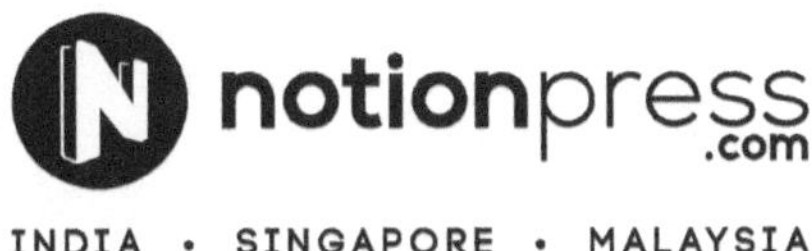

INDIA · SINGAPORE · MALAYSIA

ISBN
Paperback 979-8-89632-964-0
Hardcase 979-8-89699-371-1

I dedicate this book to my **Papaji, Mummy, Papa, Ma** and my **husband** whose unwavering support, encouragement, and belief in me have made this journey possible. I would like to thank my Guruji and Jyoti Modi without whose guidance and encouragement this book would not have been possible. This book is a reflection of all that you've given me-thank you for being a constant source of strength and inspiration.

I extend my deepest gratitude to Dr. **Mitu Kumari** for her incredible hand-made images that have brought this book to life.

Foreward

If you've ever felt that health is more than just physical well-being, *The Spiritual Dentist* by Dr. Mitu Singhal is your essential guide. This ground-breaking book uncovers the deep connections between oral health, mental well-being, and spirituality, offering a holistic perspective on dentistry and its profound impact on the mind and body.

As a Mind Performance Coach and the author of the bestseller *"Unleash the Power of Reading,"* I understand the importance of self-awareness and growth in achieving a balanced and fulfilling life. The challenges of integrating physical, emotional, and spiritual health can be daunting, but they also present opportunities for profound transformation. This book provides the insights and tools you need to recognize these connections and embrace the journey toward holistic healing and growth.

What makes *The Spiritual Dentist* truly remarkable is its ability to blend the wisdom of ancient teachings with modern practices. Drawing inspiration from the *Bhagavad Gita,* the author explores how mindfulness, conscious breathing, and compassionate care can transform the dental experience. From addressing anxiety and fear to holistic pain management, the book offers practical strategies that not only enhance oral health but also nurture the emotional and spiritual well-being of both patients and practitioners.

This book challenges us to see dentistry as more than a clinical practice—it's a healing art that connects the physical and the spiritual. It inspires readers to approach oral health as an integral part of overall wellness, reflecting the deep interconnectedness of the body, mind, and spirit.

Whether you are a dental professional, a patient, or someone curious about the intersection of health and spirituality, *The Spiritual Dentist* is a must-read. It will enlighten and empower you to embrace a more compassionate, mindful, and holistic approach to health and healing.

Best wishes,

(Dr. Manjunath M.S.)

Mind Performance Coach and Author of
"Unleash the Power of Reading

Foreward

Going through the book *"The Spiritual Dentist" made me realise that it is* a great way to understand the about the union of spirituality and dentistry. The way this book uncovers various aspects of day to day dental issues and their connections with spirituality is commendable. This book very well describes the relationship between the stress, diet control and conscious breathing with oral health and its management. Certain aspects mentioned in the book such as how dental surgeons may handle their stress can be an eye opener for many practicing young dentists. My best wishes to Dr. Mitu and I recommend everyone to read this book without fail!

Dr. Surabhi Mahidhar, MDS

Professor, Prosthodontics and Implantology

Foreward

One doesn't visit a Dentist until the pain of suffering is more than the pain of dental procedure. People tend to avoid difficult or painful interventions (like surgery) until the discomfort or pain they are experiencing becomes unbearable. But the fact is "the cure for the pain is in the pain of treatment and It is easier to resist at the beginning than at the end."

The modern dentistry is day by day becoming painless. The dentist tries best to make the treatment non-invasive if the patient comes at the initial stage of disease. Subsequently when it is intense, invasive procedures are conducted with the comfort of the patient without pain. An anaesthetic spray on the jaw prevents the pain of the prick of local Anaesthesia which further prevents the pain of the dental procedure.

The author of this book, Dr Mitu Singhal is very particular in maintaining an excellent ambience for the patient's comfort by providing a comfortable dental chair, temperature and humidity-controlled chamber with patient centric music or songs in the background. Each of these steps have been proven to be effective for patient assurance and confidence.

Beyond such arrangements, still people fear to ascend the dental chair out of "dental anxiety" or "dental phobia," in common. Several factors contribute to this fear which this book has narrated how to overcome spiritually without medication.

Bharat is a country of high ethical foundation with saints and hermitages being the source for super intellect. In course of cascaded aggressions, the links to such talents have been worn out but still it is surprising to imagine how Aarya Bhatta could find the interstellar distances without a Kepler Telescope, how Charaka developed medication for the cure of diseases, and how Sushruta developed Surgery and surgical instruments for invasive treatment of Diseases.

Dr Singhal has depicted through this book Spiritualism, in the context of dentistry, connecting the physical, emotional, and spiritual dimensions of health, suggesting that oral health is intertwined with an individual's overall well-being and spiritual state. This connection emphasizes the idea that dental conditions can be influenced by emotional and spiritual factors, and that addressing these underlying causes can lead to better health outcomes.

She has briefly blended her experience in patient treatment partially through counselling on: Mind-Body-Spirit Connection, Energy Flow and Dental Health, Chakras and Teeth, Emotional and spiritual roots of dental problems, stress management through spiritual practices, spiritual cleansing and detoxification, Box technique of pranayama for pain tolerance etc.

In her Patient-Dentist Relationship: she views her role as not just a healer of physical ailments but a supporter of the patient's overall well-being. This involves a compassionate, empathetic approach, seeing the patient as a whole being rather than just a set of dental problems.

The narrations in this book are impressive, illustrative, guiding and reassuring on pain control and dental hygiene through spiritual practices.

In reality her dental practice has most of the modern appliances and tools for dental procedures. X-rays, Dental Microscope, on screen display over wall-hung large monitor, 3-D printer for dental implant moulds, Digital Drills etc. to competently address: Hygiene and Preventive Dentistry, Restorative Dentistry, Orthodontics, Endodontics,

Periodontics, Prosthodontics, Oral and Maxillofacial Surgery, Cosmetic Dentistry etc.

A mix of Ancient Holistic strength with most modern practices will lead the Author cum Doctor to ascend success in life.

Biranchi Narayan Mahapatra

Retd. Principal Scientist, (Electronics & Instrumentation)
CRRI, ICAR.

Reviews About "The Spiritual Dentist"

This book is a remarkable step toward bridging the gap between spirituality and practical life. Too often, we forget our past mistakes and let our uncontrolled minds dictate how we face daily challenges. In such times, we need a guide—a well-wisher who stands by us through difficulties. An author is truly god-sent when they embody these values, treating their audience with kindness. This book offers such a flawless guide, bringing together professionalism and a spiritual nature to treat people with compassion.

Calming a person's fears is a role often reserved for a spiritual teacher, and Dr. Mitu Singhal's approach reflects this beautifully. Her vision of patient care is truly laudable, as she transcends caste and creed, reaching the essence of humanity and invoking divine mercy.

My heartfelt wishes to Dr. Mitu Singhal and her supportive family in this divine Endeavour.

Jai Jagannath! **A. Krishna Dasa**,
Senior Trainer/Faculty, Gita Study Circle, Puri
Gauranga Seva Foundation

I feel incredibly fortunate to have read this ground breaking book by Dr. Mitu Singhal.

It's a beautiful expression of her passion, expertise and unique perspective on dentistry and holistic well-being. This book is a remarkable exploration of the connection between oral health and inner well- being, blending modern dental science with spiritual practices, holistic pain management, and Yoga. It's a refreshing perspective that bridges the gap between physical and emotional health.

What sets this book apart is Dr. Mitu's ability to weave together scientific rigor and spiritual wisdom. The integration of Yoga, mindfulness and holistic pain management in dentistry is both innovative and inspiring. The book offers practical advice and insights for individuals and medical practitioners, this book is a treasure of knowledge. As a clinical dentist, I found Yoga topics particularly eye-opening. It not only deepened my understanding of oral health but also encouraged me to approach wellness from a more holistic perspective.

I highly recommend this book to anyone interested in holistic health, whether you are a health care professional, a patient, or simply curious about the connection between mind, body and oral health. One line that deeply resonated with me was, "Your body is a temple, but only if you treat it as one." The profound statement written in the book captures the essence of the book

Dr Mitu Kumari,
Practising Dental Surgeon,
Navi Mumbai

Dr. Mitu book Spiritual Dentist is a must read. She has taught us how important it is to discipline our self. She silently introspected worked on herself and wants to share the joy with everyone so that all can lead a healthy and happy life.

As Dr. Mitu has taken small steps made a big shift we must also take care of our physical spiritual emotional being. Take one step towards self-care the most precious gift we can give ourselves. Thank you Dr. Mitu for this insightful book which will surely help us work on ourselves

Mrs Vanjaksi,

Sadhavi

The spiritual dentist book will guide how the Teeth and Gums offers an enlightening perspective on oral health by integrating holistic principles with practical self-care techniques. The book empowers readers to take control of their dental health at home, addressing issues from gum health to detoxification.

Dr. Mitu emphasizes the connection between oral health and overall well-being, challenging conventional practices that often overlook the body's holistic nature. The guide is both informative and accessible, making it a valuable resource for anyone seeking a safer, more effective approach to dental care. This book is a must-read for those interested in merging traditional dental practices with holistic health principles.

Dr Ritu,

Practising Dental Surgeon,

Sydney, Australia

Well put together the teachings of our universal master 'Krishna'...

The commendable part is the way you are trying to integrate it in the field of work.

A spiritual dentist in the making!!

Mrs Jyoti Modi,

Devotee of Shri Sharada Math

Spirituality for most of the people can be very overwhelming and adapting its principles in daily life can be very challenging. The concept behind this book is actually very novel and unique as it tries to elucidate spirituality in a very simple yet effective manner. The manner in which the author has gelled in the principles of holistic life and aspects of Dentistry is commendable. A unique aspect about the text is the way fears and anxiety of dentists themselves are expressed, considering the fact that the author herself is a dentist. This book is a must read for the masses as well for the entire dental fraternity. I wish for the success of this amazing concept and good luck to Dr. Mitu for her future endeavours.

Dr Kunal Agarwal,

Practising Dental Surgeon

As a maxillofacial radiologist and close associate of Dr. Mitu Singhal, I have had the privilege of witnessing her transformative journey in creating The Spiritual Dentist. Knowing her both professionally and personally, I can vouch for the depth of her wisdom and the authenticity of her approach. This book transcends being a mere guide to oral health; it invites us to rethink our understanding of wellness by intertwining dentistry, mindfulness, and spiritual alignment.

Dr. Singhal's approach to oral health transcends the boundaries of conventional dentistry, embodying a profound commitment to holistic care that touches the soul. Her ability to illuminate the mouth as a portal for emotional and spiritual well-being is not only revolutionary but also deeply rooted in her unwavering belief in equality and service to humanity. Dr. Singhal's dedication to providing impeccable healthcare transcends caste, creed, and gender, reflecting her devotion to serving God through every patient she treats.

Through engaging narratives and actionable insights, she explores how oral health reflects our inner states, providing tools to address deeper imbalances. Her insights into mindful chewing, conscious breathing, and the energetic properties of food have opened my eyes to the unseen dimensions of oral care. This book has reshaped my perspective on dental wellness, encouraging me to view routine practices as sacred acts of self-care.

The universal appeal of The Spiritual Dentist is what makes it truly impactful. Whether you are a dental professional seeking a more holistic approach or someone interested in the mind-body connection, this masterpiece promises to ignite a journey of transformation. Dr. Singhal's words resonate deeply, urging us to embrace oral health not just as a physical necessity but as a pathway to harmony and healing. This book is a testament to her philosophy, reshaping the perspective of oral care into a sacred act that nurtures both body and spirit. Through her words and actions, Dr. Singhal ensures her patients receive not just exceptional care but also a transformative experience that bridges the gap between healthcare and spiritual well-being. Her work is a beacon of compassion and excellence, inspiring all to view patient care as a harmonious balance of science, empathy, and divinity.

This book is a must-read for anyone looking to integrate wellness practices into their daily life. It has left a lasting impression on me, and I am confident it will do the same for you. Don't just read this book—experience it.

Dr. Ajo Babu George,

Maxillofacial Radiologist
AI Research Scientist, IIT Kharagpur

Contents

Chapter 1

Introduction

In today's fast-paced world, health is frequently reduced to its constituent parts—our bodies are considered as distinct from our minds, and our minds are treated as separated from our spirits. Nowhere is this clearer than in dentistry, where oral health is frequently seen as separate from the rest of body. But what if I told you that your oral health is the key to not only physical wellness, but also mental clarity, emotional balance, and spiritual harmony? What if your teeth and gums are the key to a deeper, revolutionary healing journey?

This is more than just another dental care book. The Spiritual Dentist is a comprehensive examination that combines the art and science of dentistry with the knowledge of the mind-body-spirit connection. It's an opportunity to look beyond the surface of your teeth and contemplate how the care you provide your mouth can have an impact on all aspects of your life. When we adjust our perspective, dentistry becomes more than just fillings and cleanings; it is about growing awareness, releasing trauma, and tapping into the body's natural ability to heal itself.

Whether you're a seasoned dentist wishing to strengthen the bond between your office and your patients, or someone looking to improve your overall health and well-being, this book is intended to change the way you see your mouth—and, by extension, your entire existence. This guide will teach you how to balance your oral health with your physical, emotional, and spiritual needs, as well as how to establish a daily dental care routine that nourishes not only your smile but also your soul.

The Forgotten Connection: Mind, Body, and Mouth.

Many of us have been trained to think of our mouths as distinct from the rest of our bodies. We go to the dentist for regular cleanings, cavities, and cosmetic adjustments. Rarely do we consider how our dental health affects our emotional or spiritual well-being. The mouth is one of the most sensitive and linked organs in the body. It is a direct route for expression, digestion, and communication that plays an important part in how we perceive the world.

When something goes wrong in the mouth, whether it's tooth decay, gum disease, or jaw pain, it typically reflects deeper internal imbalances. Stress, worry, and unresolved emotions are typically manifested in oral disorders ranging from teeth grinding to canker sores (also known as Apthous ulcers). In contrast, repairing the mouth can reveal hidden reserves of vitality, clarity, and emotional resilience.

As a dentist, I've spent years studying and practicing the technical aspects of dental health, but it wasn't until I adopted a holistic approach that I realized the mouth's true significance. My path has taught me that repairing the oral cavity can lead to emotional freedom, energetic balance, and spiritual progress. Your smile is more than simply a reflection of good hygiene; it is a doorway into your inner world.

Your Invitation for Transformation

This book is more than just theory; it is about practical transformation. You'll find tools, activities, and insights to help you better understand your mouth and the communications it sends you. You'll learn how to incorporate mindfulness into your dental routine, how to relieve emotional stress in the jaw, and how to nourish your body holistically with correct oral care.

By the end of this voyage, you will understand that caring for your teeth is a sacred act. Whether you're a dentist, a health buff, or just curious about the mind-body link, The Spiritual Dentist will reveal the significant influence your mouth has on your total well-being.

Are you prepared to embark on a journey to uncover the hidden link between your oral health and your spirituality? Let us take the first step together.

Holistic health connects dentistry and spirituality by acknowledging that oral health is inextricably linked to overall mental, physical, and spiritual well-being. While traditional dentistry frequently focuses primarily on the physical aspects—teeth, gums, and bones—holistic dentistry delves further, investigating how emotional, energy, and even spiritual imbalances can emerge in the mouth. This technique does more than just repair cavities and misaligned teeth; it views the mouth as a portal to total wellness, revealing the subtle information our oral health conveys about our deeper state of being.

Consider the scenario of a patient with chronic teeth grinding (bruxism). In traditional dentistry, this could be addressed with a mouthguard or full mouth rehabilitation. However, the dentist takes a holistic approach, investigating the emotional and spiritual origins of this illness. Teeth grinding is commonly associated with stress, unresolved anger, or a sense of being out of sync with one's life purpose. By treating the underlying cause—whether through mindfulness, meditation, or even energy healing—the patient not only relieves the grinding but also gains emotional and spiritual release, resulting in a profound sense of serenity and harmony. By saying this, I am not denigrating current dental treatment methods; rather, a holistic approach can be a helpful supplement to them.

This is where dentistry meets spirituality. The mouth is the body's entrance to expression; holding back unspoken words or emotional suffering can result in dental difficulties. Holistic dentistry becomes a road toward full-body harmony by mending the body while also embracing the emotional and spiritual aspects of wellness. The link is obvious: mending the mouth can lead to healing the mind and soul, transforming dental treatment into an effective tool for personal development and spiritual enlightenment.

Motivation for Writing This Book.

My journey as a dentist has been more than simply a professional one; it has been a profound spiritual revelation. For many years, I practiced traditional dentistry, focusing on the technical aspects of oral health, operations, and frequent tooth issues. But, over time, I began to sense something deeper, something that went beyond the physical reality of the mouth, teeth, and gum. There was a deeper relationship at work—a link between dental health and an individual's emotional, mental, and spiritual wellness.

As I became more involved with spirituality, I discovered that the mouth, the entryway to expression, digestion, and communication, possesses enormous power that extends far beyond its biological purpose. As I studied mindfulness, energy work, and holistic treatment, it became evident that dental health is inextricably linked to the entire human experience—mind, body, and spirit. This insight changed the way I performed dentistry, changing it into a holistic art form in which dental care became a vehicle for deep healing.

One scenario comes to me that exemplifies this powerful link. A patient came to me with chronic ulcers. Despite following the best treatment regimens, including Laser therapy and topical medicines, the problem remained. Beyond this, there was no conventional treatment left to offer the patient, therefore she did not receive any relief. What was the cause of the ulcers? Why was the patient not obtaining relief?

This puzzled both of us. As we dug further, I realized that this patient was carrying significant emotional burdens—grief and unprocessed trauma from the recent loss of a loved one to oral cancer. I began incorporating mindfulness practices into her treatment, urging her to tune into her emotions and understand how they were expressing in her body, particularly her mouth.

We worked on stress-reduction tactics and emotional release exercises together, and her ulcers improved as well as her emotional well-being over time. What had been a chronic physical problem was alleviated after the emotional impediments were removed. This was just one of several experiences that solidified my opinion that dental health is inextricably linked to mental and spiritual wellness. Healing the mouth can often release imprisoned emotions, trauma, and spiritual imbalances.

This wasn't a solitary incident. I began to see emotional trends in individuals with Temporomandibular Disorders (TMDs), including suppressed anger, bruxism, stress, and misalignment with life purpose. It became evident that the mouth served as a mirror, reflecting what was going on in the deeper layers of the psyche. So I began incorporating spiritual practices, such as mindfulness and meditation, into my dental treatments. I discovered that when patients regarded oral care as a sacred act—an opportunity to nourish both their bodies and spirits—the effects were transformational. They noticed not only changes in their dental health, but also in their emotional balance and spiritual clarity.

This journey prompted me to write The Spiritual Dentist. I felt compelled to share these insights with both the dentistry community and the general public. We live in a world where health is frequently segmented, with dentistry perceived as a strictly physical science. But

I believe it's time for a paradigm shift, one that recognizes the mouth's critical role in our overall health. By combining spirituality and dental care, we can achieve a higher degree of healing—one that addresses the whole person rather than simply their symptoms.

My purpose in publishing this book is to spark fresh conversations about the importance of oral health in overall well-being. I want to encourage both dentists and patients to see the mouth as more than just a collection of teeth and gums, but as an important element of our emotional, mental, and spiritual health. The link between dentistry and spirituality may appear unusual, but my clinical experiences have shown me that it is not only genuine, but transformative.

I've seen patients become more attentive of their dental treatment, utilizing it as a time to reflect on their mental state, relationships, and life's purpose. I've seen the remarkable release that occurs when patients are encouraged to grasp the underlying causes of their oral issues—whether it's an accumulation of unresolved sadness, hidden truths, or buried anger. And I've seen their oral health improve alongside their mental and spiritual health, demonstrating that this holistic approach has the potential to cure on numerous levels.

My hope is that by sharing my experiences, stories, and thoughts, you will begin to see your dental health as an important component of your total wellness, and that you will embrace the idea that true healing requires addressing the mind, body, and spirit all at once. This book is an invitation to join me on a voyage of discovery, where dental care can lead to better wholeness, balance, and peace.

Chapter 2

Oral Health as a Reflection of Inner Well-Being

Our oral health is more than just a biological sign; it also reflects our overall well-being. It has a deeper relationship to the mind and spirit, showing far more than cavities or gum disease. Our emotional, mental, and spiritual moods are frequently reflected in the appearance of our teeth, gums, and oral surroundings. A healthy smile is more than just a result of proper oral care; it also indicates inner tranquillity.

When our emotions are out of balance, our mouths frequently carry the brunt of the load. Take stress as an example. Chronic stress can appear in a variety of ways across the body, including the mouth. Teeth grinding, or bruxism, is a frequent reaction to unresolved stress and anxiety. Many people grind their teeth while sleeping, entirely oblivious of the damage they are causing to their teeth and tmj (temporomandibular joint). The act of grinding is more than just a physical movement; it is a symbolic reflection of the internal pressure we carry. Our bodies reflect our challenges, and the mouth, as such an intimate part of our daily life, expresses these conflicts openly.

Emotions like grief, rage, and joy have an impact on our oral health. Individuals who are extremely worried may develop chronic dry mouth because stress suppresses the salivary glands. A lack of saliva creates an environment in which bacteria can grow, resulting in cavities, gum disease, foul breath, and fungal infections such as oral candidiasis on various mucosal surfaces. In contrast, joy and a sense of tranquility frequently urge us to maintain our general health, including oral care. When we are happy and balanced, we are more inclined to take care of ourselves holistically, such as brushing, flossing, and having regular dental examinations.

Teeth as symbols of personal power and self-reflection

Beyond the mental and emotional ties, our spiritual well-being has an impact on our oral health. Spiritual imbalance or dissociation can show as bodily symptoms, such as oral problems. Many holistic practitioners think that our teeth and gums are connected to the body's energy systems, known as meridians or chakras. If we are spiritually out of alignment, particular parts of our tongue may develop difficulties. For example, unresolved personal concerns or a lack of purpose may be energetically aligned with dental complications. Each tooth is thought to correspond to a distinct organ or mental condition, implying that oral health may be an entry point for comprehending deeper, unresolved spiritual issues.

In ancient Ayurvedic practice, the mouth is regarded as an important location of cleansing and energy movement. The technique of oil pulling, which involves swishing oil around the mouth to draw out impurities, reflects the concept that the mouth has important connections to our general health. This is more than just a cleansing ritual; it's a technique to bring balance to the physical body and the energetic systems that sustain it. A spiritually fed person frequently has a healthier oral environment, as the balance obtained via meditation, mindfulness, and connection with higher consciousness affects all aspects of their physical being. I'd like to emphasize again that this is not a substitute for brushing, but rather a useful supplement.

The meals we eat also reflect our emotional and spiritual situations. When we are emotionally distressed, we prefer to eat more comfort foods, particularly sweet or processed ones. These foods have an instant impact on both our bodily and oral health, causing tooth caries. Our nutritional choices frequently reflect our emotional demands. When we are detached from ourselves or coping with unresolved emotions, we may turn to these foods for consolation, perpetuating a cycle of poor oral and overall health.

Mindfulness is an effective way to bridge the gap between oral health and overall well-being. When done with focus, even something as basic as brushing your teeth can become a moment of meditation. When we approach oral care with mindfulness, we are not just cleaning our teeth; we are also strengthening the bond between our inner state and our physical body. Each brushstroke can serve as a reminder to practice self-care, which includes both physical and spiritual well-being. This mindful approach encourages us to slow down, appreciate self-care, and focus on our emotional and mental states.

Practitioners can identify internal abnormalities by evaluating the color, texture, and shape of the tongue. A bloated or pale tongue, for example, may suggest digestive problems, low iron levels (anaemia), or poor energy flow, whereas deep fractures may indicate chronic dehydration or emotional stress. Psychosomatic illnesses such as Lichen Planus can produce substantial ulcerations in the tongue, resulting in a burning sensation and making eating difficult. A cascade of events is started, which eventually leads to the patient's nutrition being impaired. This emphasizes the notion that the mouth is a direct reflection of our interior well-being, providing cues about what we may need to address emotionally or spiritually. Finally, dental health is more than simply a surface-level concern; it is inextricably linked to our total wellness. Our emotions, mental clarity, and spiritual harmony all influence the health of our mouths. Understanding this connection allows us to approach dental care not as a standalone profession, but as part of a comprehensive approach to wellness. Taking care of our mouth is an act of self-love and contemplation that benefits not only our physical health but also our emotional and spiritual well-being. A healthy grin, viewed through this perspective, is more than just an aesthetic triumph; it is a shining mirror of inner harmony and balance.

Teeth are more than just tools for eating and breaking down food; they are powerful symbols of human strength and self-expression. Throughout history, cultures have viewed teeth as symbols of strength, vitality, and personal identity.

Tongue's Relationship to Communication and Truth

Bhagavad Gita, Chapter 17, Verse 15:

> *"Anudvegakaraṃ vākyaṃ satyaṃ priyahitaṃ ca*
> *yatsvādhyāyābhyasanam caiva vāṅmayaṃ tapa ucyate"*

Translation: "Austerity of speech consists in speaking words that are truthful, pleasing, beneficial, and not agitating to others, and also in regularly reciting the Vedic scriptures."

This passage emphasizes the significance of using the tongue for genuine and constructive communication, connecting speech with dharma, and caring about the well-being of others.

Throughout history and across cultures, the tongue has been associated with the expression of truth, honesty, and the power of words. To truly understand the profound connection between the tongue, communication, and truth, let us explore this idea visually and through impactful examples that resonate deeply. The ability to communicate one's truth is one of the most powerful manifestations of personal power. Imagine a powerful orator standing in front of an audience, his tongue—the key tool of communication—shaping words that can inspire revolutions or bring peace. The tongue gives form to thoughts, translating the intangible into the spoken word, influencing minds, and shifting perspectives.

Physiology and Communication

The tongue's intricate muscle network allows for a wide range of speech sounds, and its flexibility and agility enable us to form complex words and expressions. Damage to the tongue, whether through injury, disease, or neurological disorders like aphasia, can hinder one's ability to speak clearly, emphasizing the tongue's deep connection with effective communication. Speech therapy, for example, frequently focuses on retraining the tongue to regain articulation and fluency in individuals recovering from a stroke that affects speech. Exercises like tongue movements and strengthening techniques help restore communication abilities, emphasizing the tongue's importance.

Symbolic Role: Speaking the Truth

Across many cultures and spiritual traditions, the tongue represents the expression of truth. The phrase "speaking with a forked tongue" refers to someone being deceitful, implying that when used in alignment with higher principles, the tongue conveys honesty and authenticity. In many ways, controlling the tongue becomes a spiritual practice, guiding us to align our communication with our deepest truths. In ancient Vedic teachings, the tongue is associated with the concept of Satya (truth), and in Buddhism, the practice of Right Speech encourages using the tongue to speak words that are truthful, kind, and constructive. In a dental practice, for example, if a patient is afraid or anxious about a procedure, the dentist's calm and truthful communication, powered by the tongue, can alleviate the patient's concerns. A simple, honest explanation can build trust, transforming the dentist-patient interaction into a spiritual exchange based on truth.

Tongue and Personal Integrity

On a more personal level, the tongue acts as a mirror of our inner integrity. When we are mindful of what we say and how we say it, our words carry more weight and sincerity, reflecting our own alignment with truth. For example, a person who practices mindful speaking may pause before responding in a stressful conversation, engaging the tongue to express only what is necessary and truthful, avoiding unnecessary conflict and fostering deeper connections.

Gandhi's Communication Through Nonviolence:

Mahatma Gandhi's speech was a reflection of his inner beliefs, embodying the idea that truth ("Satya") and nonviolence ("Ahimsa") are intertwined. Gandhi's words, though soft and often quiet, conveyed a powerful message of peace and resistance to oppression, demonstrating how the tongue, when used with truth and integrity, can lead movements and change the course of history.

To summarize, the tongue is more than simply a physical organ for taste and speaking; it is a portal to communicating our inner truths and keeping integrity in our interactions. By becoming aware of how we utilize our tongues, we may improve both our communication and spiritual progress.

Key takeaways:

- Oral health is a reflection of inner well-being.
- Our dental health, specifically our teeth and gums, reflects our emotional, mental, and spiritual status.
- Stress, worry, and spiritual imbalance can cause concerns such as tooth grinding, dry mouth, and gum disease.
- A balanced inner life fosters healthy oral habits and general well-being.

- Mindful oral care, such as brushing and flossing with focus, can promote both physical health and emotional serenity.

- Teeth are symbols of personal power and self-expression.

- Teeth represent strength, tenacity, and personal power, which influences how we present ourselves.

- Grinding teeth or ignoring oral hygiene can indicate tension or suppressed emotions, whereas a bright smile expresses confidence and self-esteem.

- Throughout history, teeth have been altered or ornamented to represent personal identity and status.

- Restoring or improving one's grin can lead to a stronger sense of empowerment and self-expression.

- The Tongue: Its Relationship to Communication and Truth

- The tongue is essential for communication, Moulding the words that communicate our inner reality.

- Ancient rituals linked the state of the tongue to both physical and mental health, with a healthy tongue representing clarity and transparency.

- Truth-telling through speech empowers people and fosters trust, whereas silence or suppressed speech might represent internal turmoil or fear.

Chapter 3

Conscious Breathing and Oral Health

This chapter delves into the relationship between conscious breathing and dental health. Although we breathe unconsciously every day, the way we breathe can have a significant impact on our overall health, including our oral health. Conscious breathing is the practice of being aware of and deliberately controlling one's breath.

The relationship between breathing and oral health

When we think about breathing, we often think about how it affects our lungs and cardiovascular system. However, every breath begins in the mouth, and the quality of that breath can affect oral health in several important ways. The way we breathe—through our nose or mouth—plays a critical role in maintaining the delicate balance of oral hygiene, moisture, and proper jaw alignment.

1. Nasal vs Mouth Breathing

   Nasal breathing is the most natural and optimal way for humans to take in air. Nasal breathing helps filter out dust, allergens, and other particles, while also warming and humidifying the air before it reaches the lungs. More importantly for oral health, nasal breathing helps maintain moisture levels in the mouth and encourages proper tongue posture. This reduces the risk of developing dry mouth (xerostomia), which can lead to increased bacterial growth and bad breath. Mouth breathing, on the other hand, can have a negative impact on oral health because it causes the mouth to dry out, making saliva less effective in neutralizing acids and washing away food particles. As a result, mouth breathers are more likely to develop cavities, gum disease, and even misaligned teeth due to altered tongue and jaw posture.

2. Oxygenation & Healing

Deep, diaphragmatic breathing increases oxygen supply to the gums and soft tissues of the mouth, promoting faster healing from dental procedures or gum inflammation. Conversely, shallow, rapid breathing depletes the body of oxygen, slowing the healing process and impairing immune function.

The Impact of Stress and Breath on Dental Health

Stress is a significant factor in both general health and dental wellness. When we are stressed, we often fall into shallow, rapid breathing patterns, which activate the body's fight-or-flight response. This can lead to a cascade of negative effects on the mouth and teeth, including jaw clenching, teeth grinding (bruxism), and an increased susceptibility to gum disease.

Slow, deep breathing can help reduce stress and its negative impact on oral health. By shifting from the stress-inducing sympathetic nervous system to the calming parasympathetic nervous system, we can not only relax the body but also protect our teeth from stress-related damage, such as grinding and clenching, which can wear down enamel and strain the jaw muscles.

Conscious Breathing Practices for Dental Health

Incorporating mindful breathing exercises into everyday routines can enhance both your overall health and your oral health. Here are some simple ways to practice at home:

- **Diaphragmatic Breathing**: Place one hand on your chest and the other on your abdomen. Inhale deeply through your nose, allowing your abdomen to rise while keeping your chest still. Exhale slowly through your nose, feeling your abdomen fall. Do this for 5-10 minutes every day to promote relaxation and oxygenation.

- **Box Breathing**: Inhale through your nose for four counts, hold your breath for four, expel for four, and hold again for four. This rhythmic breathing helps regulate your nervous system, reduce stress, and promotes healing in the body.

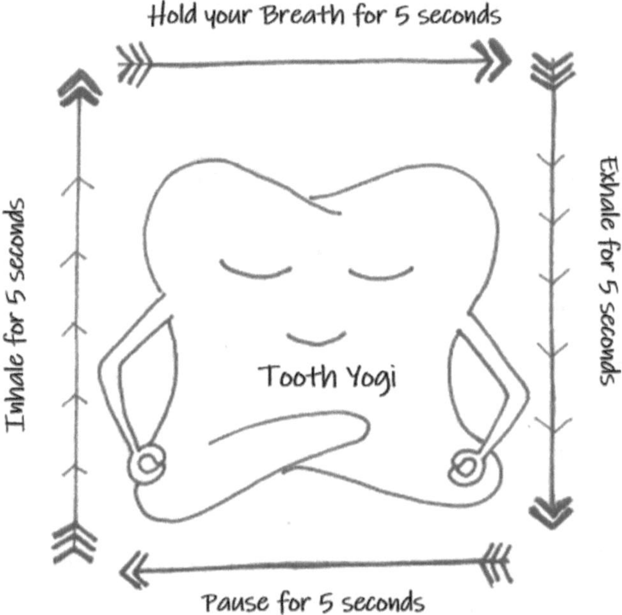

- **Alternate Nostril Breathing (Nadi Shodhana)** involves closing your right nostril with your thumb and inhaling deeply through your left nostril, then closing your left nostril with your finger and exhaling through your right nostril. This technique balances the body's energy and improves respiratory function, which contributes to overall wellness, including oral health.

Conscious breathing is more than just a tool for calming the mind; it's a practice that supports the health of your entire body, including your oral health. By promoting proper oxygenation, reducing stress, and encouraging nasal breathing, mindful breathing techniques can protect against cavities, gum disease, and other dental issues. Incorporating these simple but powerful practices into your daily routine will contribute to a healthy, vibrant smile and a sense of calmness.

In the coming chapters, we will look at more integrative practices that bridge the gap between traditional dentistry and holistic health, as we continue our journey toward total dental wellness for the mind, body, and spirit.

Diseases and Conditions Caused By Mouth Breathing

Mouth breathing can cause a variety of oral health difficulties because it affects moisture levels in the oral cavity, airflow dynamics, and overall oral physiology. The diseases and ailments caused by mouth breathing are listed below, along with technical jargon and explanations.

1. Xerostomia (dry mouth)

   Mouth breathing causes excessive saliva evaporation, which reduces the natural moisture in the oral cavity. Saliva is essential for maintaining oral hygiene because it buffers acids, washes away food particles, and protects oral tissues.

   Pathophysiology: When the mouth is always open, the protective barrier of saliva is disrupted, allowing germs and plaque to collect, increasing the risk of various oral disorders such dental caries and periodontal disease.

   Symptoms:
   - Dry sensation in the mouth.
   - Thick, sticky saliva.

- Difficulty swallowing, burning sensation on eating
- Frequent thirst.

2. Dental caries (Cavities)

Xerostomia, induced by mouth breathing, lowers saliva, which normally helps maintain an ideal pH in the mouth. When saliva is diminished, bacterial activity increases, resulting to demineralization of tooth enamel and the development of caries. When mouth breathing reduces salivary flow, acids produced by cariogenic bacteria like Streptococcus mutans remain on tooth surfaces for longer periods of time, causing demineralization. These demineralized areas eventually progress to cavitated lesions, where the hard enamel is lost and the softer dentin is exposed, resulting in tooth decay.

Symptoms:

- Chalky white patches on teeth (initial caries lesions).
- Cavities or holes in teeth
- Sensitivity to hot, cold, or sweet food
- Pain from eating or biting

3. Gingivitis (gum inflammation)

Mouth breathing can dry out the gums, causing discomfort and an increased risk of inflammation. A dry oral environment promotes bacterial proliferation, especially around the gingival edges, which leads to gingivitis. Gingivitis, if left untreated, can proceed to periodontitis because the bacterial toxins in plaque cause an immunological response, resulting in inflammation, swelling, and bleeding at the gingival borders.

Symptoms:

- Red, swollen, or sensitive gums.

- Bleeding while brushing and flossing
- Bad breath.
- Gum recession in severe situations.

4. Periodontitis (advanced gum disease).

Periodontitis, a more severe form of gum disease in which the supporting elements of the teeth, such as the alveolar bone and periodontal ligaments, are destroyed, can develop from prolonged xerostomia and untreated gingivitis caused by mouth breathing.

Pathophysiology: Bacterial plaque causes chronic inflammation at the gumline, which spreads deeper into the periodontal tissues. The immune system's response to the bacterial biofilm destroys the periodontal ligament and alveolar bone, resulting in pocket formation, gum recession, and tooth mobility or loss.

Symptoms:

- Deep periodontal pockets.
- gingival recession
- Loose or missing teeth
- Consistent foul breath and unpleasant taste

5. Halitosis (chronic bad breath).

Halitosis can be caused by xerostomia and bacterial overgrowth in the mouth. When the mouth is dry, bacteria that create volatile sulfur compounds (VSCs) thrive, which contributes to bad breath.

Pathophysiology: Reduced salivary flow impairs the natural cleansing of food particles and dead cells, promoting the growth of anaerobic bacteria, particularly Porphyromonas gingivalis and Prevotella intermedia, which produce foul-smelling sulfur compounds like hydrogen sulfide and methyl mercaptan.

Symptoms:

- Persistent bad breath, even after brushing and using mouthwash.
- Dry, sticky mouth.
- Coating of the tongue or throat.
- Metallic flavor in the mouth.

6. Malocclusion (misalignment of the teeth and jaw)

Malocclusion

Chronic mouth breathing during early childhood can disrupt normal jaw and dental development, causing alterations in tongue location and altered jaw growth patterns, ultimately leading to malocclusion (improper tooth alignment). Mouth breathing causes the tongue to rest lower in the oral cavity rather than against the palate, which is its natural position. This lack of upward pressure on the maxilla (upper jaw) during development can cause it to become narrow and high-arched. Additionally, the mandible (lower jaw) may become retruded (pulled back), resulting in a class II malocclusion (overbite) or other bite discrepancies.

Symptoms:

- Crowded or crooked teeth.
- Narrow palate.
- Open bite or crossbite?
- Facial asymmetry.

7. Sleep Apnea (Obstructive Sleep Apnea—OSA)

Mouth breathing, particularly during sleep, is a risk factor for obstructive sleep apnea (OSA), a disorder in which the airway becomes clogged, resulting in disrupted breathing during sleep. Chronic mouth breathing can cause the tissues of the airway to collapse more readily. Obstructive sleep apnea (OSA) is a condition in which the soft tissues in the throat relax, obstructing the airway and causing repeated arousals from sleep. During sleep, mouth breathing reduces the tone of the muscles in the upper airway, resulting in increased airway resistance and collapse. OSA is linked to a higher risk of cardiovascular disease, fatigue during the day, and cognitive impairment.

Symptoms:

- Loud snoring
- interrupted breathing during sleep.
- Daytime sleepiness or tiredness.
- Upon waking, I had a dry mouth and aching throat.

8. Enamel Erosion.

   Enamel erosion can be accelerated by mouth breathing due to dry mouth and greater exposure to acidic circumstances. When saliva's protective buffering ability is lost, teeth become more exposed to the effects of food acids and bacterial byproducts. Enamel erosion weakens teeth, making them more prone to sensitivity and decay. Saliva plays an important role in buffering oral pH and remineralizing tooth enamel. When saliva levels drop, teeth become more vulnerable to erosion from acidic foods, beverages, and stomach acid (in cases of gastroesophageal reflux disease).

Symptoms:

- Increased dental sensitivity, particularly to cold or acidic foods.
- Yellowing of teeth as the enamel thins, exposing the underlying dentin

- The teeth have rounded, smooth edges.
- Surface wear on the teeth, resulting in chipping or fractures

Pranayama and Its Role in Holistic Dental Care

Bhagavad Gita, Chapter 4, Verse 29.

"apāne juhvati prāṇaṁ prāṇe 'pānaṁ tathāpare
prāṇāpāna-gatī ruddhvā prāṇāyāma-parāyaṇāḥ."

अपाने जुह्वति प्राणं प्राणेऽपानं तथापरे |
प्राणापानगती रुद्ध्वा प्राणायामपरायणाः

Translation: "Others offer the outgoing breath into the incoming, and the incoming into the outgoing, thus practicing breath control. They are intent on the regulation of the life breath."

This stanza addresses the ancient yogic practice of *Pranayama*, which involves intentionally regulating one's breath. The Sanskrit word *pranayama* is composed of two parts. *"Prana"* translates as breath, vigor, energy, power, vital energy or life force. Prana is the subtle energy that flows through the body in nadis or energy channels. These pathways move and circulate prana throughout the entire body. *"Yama"* translates to control, restraint, regulation, or discipline. Concept of pranayama emphasizes attentive control over breathing, which is linked to practices that enhance overall health, including dental wellness.

Links to Oral Health:

Conscious breathing, as part of pranayama, reduces stress and can improve systemic health. This has a direct impact on oral health because stress is often linked to conditions like bruxism (teeth grinding), gum disease, and dry mouth. You can draw on this connection to explain how the Gita emphasizes breath awareness, which promotes a calm state that benefits the mouth, teeth, and gums. Pranayama, the ancient practice of controlled, mindful breathing, plays a transformative role in holistic wellness, including oral health. Pranayama encompasses a variety of breath-control techniques designed to harmonize the mind, body, and spirit. Though traditionally known for its effects on mental clarity and respiratory function, pranayama can also have profound benefits.

Physiology of Pranayama and Oral Health

Several pranayama techniques, particularly diaphragmatic breathing, promote deeper inhalations and slower exhalations, which improve cardiovascular function and enhance the delivery of oxygenated blood to oral tissues.

Furthermore, pranayama encourages nasal breathing—the optimal breathing method for oral health. Nasal breathing filters, humidifies, and warms the air before it enters the lungs, reducing the risk of xerostomia (dry mouth) and the subsequent development of oral diseases such as dental caries and periodontal disease. Mouth breathing, a common habit in individuals with respiratory difficulties, can disrupt the balance of oral microbiota and lead to bacterial overgrowth.

Stress Reduction and its Effect on Oral Health.

Pranayama is a powerful tool for managing stress, which plays a critical role in the etiology of many oral conditions. Chronic stress can manifest in bruxism (teeth grinding), temporomandibular joint disorder (TMD), and oral mucosal lesions. The practice of pranayama activates the parasympathetic nervous system, triggering the body's relaxation response. This shift from sympathetic dominance reduces muscle tension in the jaw and face, mitigating the risk of stress-related

Pranayama reduces the body's production of cortisol, a stress hormone that can impair immune function and exacerbate inflammation in the gums, contributing to periodontitis. Regular pranayama practice helps restore the body's homeostatic balance, allowing the immune system to function more effectively in protecting oral tissues from pathogenic microorganisms.

Pranayama Techniques for Oral Health

Specific pranayama techniques can be adapted to improve many elements of oral health and general wellness. Here are some effective pranayama practices that offer direct and indirect advantages for the mouth, gums, and overall dental well-being.

Nadi Shodhana (Alternate Nostril Breathing):

This balancing technique helps regulate the flow of energy (prana) throughout the body, enhancing respiratory function and promoting nasal breathing. By facilitating better airflow through the nasal passages, Nadi Shodhana reduces mouth breathing, preventing dryness and bacterial imbalances associated with xerostomia.

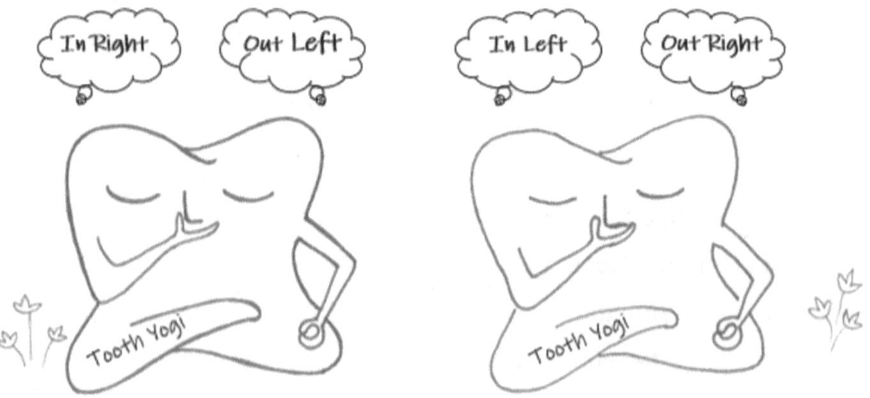

Bhramari (Bee Breath):

This pranayama is known for its calming effects on the nervous system. The gentle humming vibrations created during exhalation stimulate the vagus nerve, activating parasympathetic pathways that relieve stress and tension in the face, jaw, and neck. It's especially useful for reducing bruxism and TMJ-related discomfort.

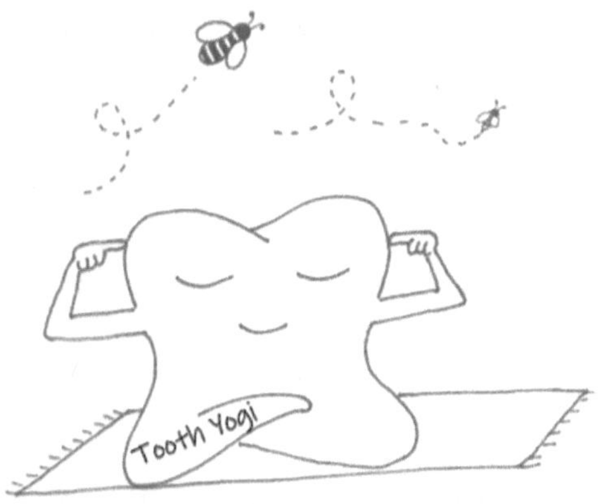

Ujjayi (Victorious Breath) pranayama:

It is characterized by a soft constriction at the back of the throat, improves oxygenation and promotes relaxation. This practice enhances the body's ability to recover from oral surgery or periodontal procedures by boosting tissue repair via increased oxygen supply to the oral cavity.

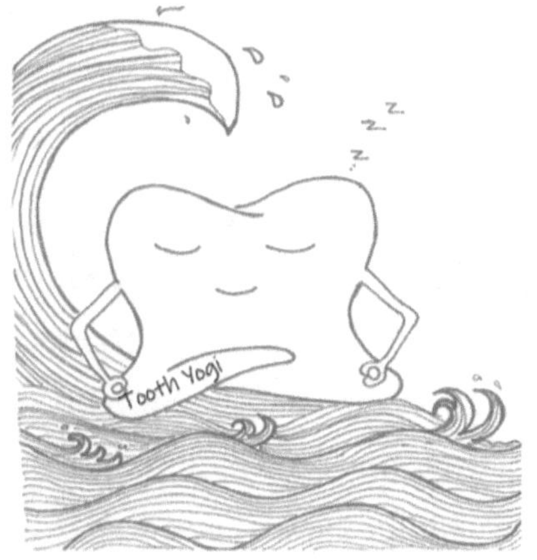

Kapalabhati (Skull Shining Breath)

This technique that detoxifies the body by expelling stale air and boosting lymphatic drainage, while also supporting the immune system and preventing oral infections like oral candidiasis.

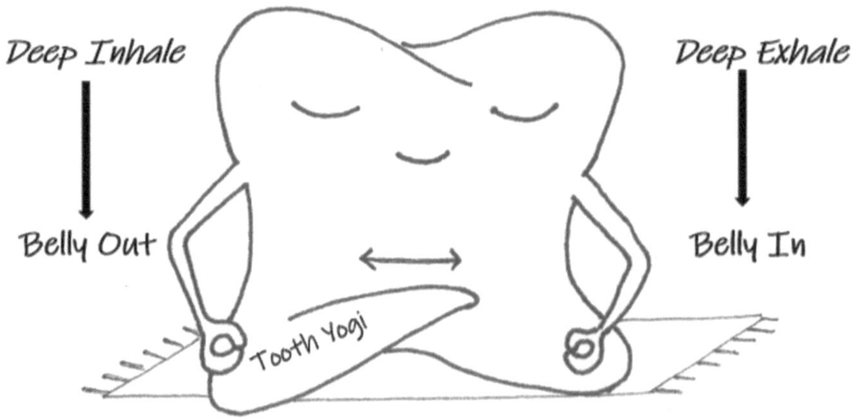

The Energetic and Holistic Dimensions of Pranayama in Oral Care

According to yogic philosophy, the mouth is a part of the vishuddha chakra (throat chakra), which governs communication, purification, and expression. A balanced throat chakra is associated with clear communication and self-expression, while A balanced throat chakra is associated with clear communication and self-expression, while an imbalance can manifest as oral health issues such as sore throat, gum infections, and bad breath (halitosis).

Pranayama, or controlled breathing, helps to unblock energy pathways (nadis) associated with the throat chakra, promoting not only physical healing but also emotional and energetic purification. Regular pranayama practice supports the alignment and function of the vishuddha chakra, promoting the integrity of the mouth, gums, and surrounding tissues on both physical and subtle levels.

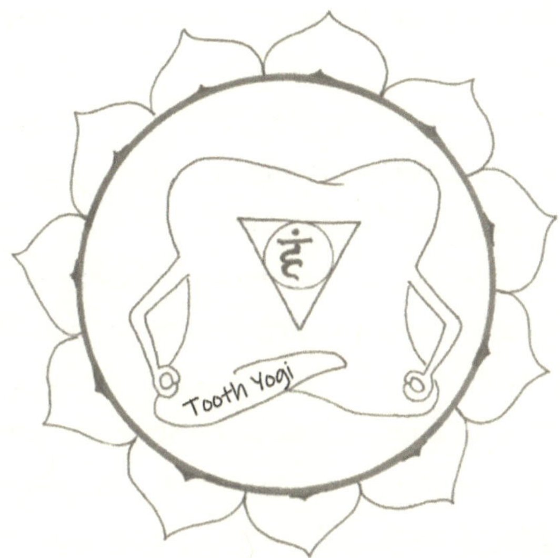

Key Points: Conscious Breathing and Oral Health

- Breathing and Oral Health: Conscious breathing, particularly nasal breathing, is critical for maintaining oral moisture and preventing dry mouth, which can contribute to dental issues such as cavities, gum disease, and poor breath.

- Pranayama's Role in Oral Care: Pranayama, or attentive breathing, promotes oral health by increasing oxygen flow, lowering stress, and encouraging appropriate nasal breathing, all of which help to prevent mouth disorders.

- Dry Mouth Prevention: Nasal breathing maintains appropriate saliva production, protecting the mouth from dangerous microorganisms and promoting a healthy oral environment.

- Pranayama reduces stress and cortisol levels, which reduces the risk of gum disease and other stress-induced oral diseases such as bruxism.

- Nasal breathing filters and humidifies the air, lowering the incidence of dry mouth and its accompanying hazards, whereas mouth breathing causes a dry oral environment and bacterial imbalances.

- Pranayama promotes holistic health by balancing the body's energies, particularly the throat chakra, which is associated with speech and self-expression.

- Effective Pranayama Techniques: Practices like as Nadi Shodhana (Alternate Nostril Breathing) and Bhramari (Bee Breath) help to alleviate tension, promote healthy jaw alignment, and improve oral and respiratory health.

- Pranayama improves oral wellness and general health by bringing mind, body, and spirit into harmony.

Chapter 4

Mindful Eating May Nourish the Mouth, Body, and Spirit

Mindful eating is a transformative experience that connects the mind, body, and spirit. It is the art of being fully present while eating, understanding the energy exchange that occurs between the eater and the food, and appreciating the act of nourishment. "Your body is a temple, but only if you treat it as one." This quote by Astrid Alauda rings especially true in the context of mindful eating. Every bite you take is an opportunity to respect your body and provide it with what it truly needs. In dentistry, the mouth becomes the first sacred point of contact with food—what we choose to put in our mouth affects not only our physical health but also our emotional and spiritual balance.

When you eat mindfully, you slow down, allowing yourself to savor every texture, flavor, and aroma. This seemingly simple act of awareness can radically shift your relationship with food.

The ancient Ayurvedic proverb "Chew your drink, and drink your food" emphasizes the significance of this practice. The act of chewing, for example, stimulates neural activity that aids in the processing of emotions. By engaging all of the senses, the brain can receive signals that calm the body and mind. From a nutritional standpoint, mindful eating is also about the conscious selection of food. Food can be medicine, and what we eat has a direct impact on our oral health. A patient who came to me with severe gum inflammation realized that her diet, which was high in processed foods and sugar, was exacerbating her condition. When she became more mindful of her choices—opting for fresh, whole foods rich in vitamins and minerals—her oral health dramatically improved.

Eating with gratitude transforms the experience into a spiritual practice. It's about acknowledging where the food comes from, the effort that went into growing and preparing it, and the nourishment it provides. When we eat with gratitude, we're more likely to make healthier choices that benefit not only our teeth but our entire being. One day in my clinic, I asked a patient, "When was the last time you truly tasted your food?" She paused and realized she was eating

On the other hand, when we eat mindlessly, especially when we eat highly processed foods loaded with sugar, we disconnect from our bodies. We may be eating to satisfy a temporary craving, but it often comes at the expense of our long-term health. Sugar, the leading cause of tooth decay, not only erodes enamel but also dulls our senses. It's no surprise that those who are more mindful of their food choices have better dental health.

Bulimia Nervosa, which can cause significant enamel loss owing to frequent forceful vomiting, is a condition in which people use food as a source of comfort when they are worried, anxious, or upset.

Mindful eating can have a direct impact on oral health, particularly when the food of choice is sugary or processed. I've had patients who experienced tooth decay, not because they weren't brushing or flossing, but because they were relying on sweets during emotional upheavals. When they began practicing mindful eating, they started recognizing their emotional triggers, reaching for healthier options, and saw remarkable improvements in both their mental and dental health

The journey of mindful eating is not just about the food on your plate; it's about cultivating a deeper relationship with your body, understanding the signals it sends, and honoring the act of nourishment. When we approach food with respect and awareness, we elevate it from a mere necessity to a sacred ritual, and we care for our teeth and overall well-being.

The energetic influence of food

"The food you eat can be either the safest and most powerful form of medicine or the slowest form of poison," says Ann Wigmore, the raw food movement's pioneer.

Food is more than simply calories or nutrition; it contains energetic vibrations that influence not only the physical body but also the mind and spirit. Food's energetic impact is a concept that has its roots in ancient wisdom as well as modern holistic approaches. In essence, everything we consume has a unique vibrational frequency that interacts with our body's energy fields, influencing how we feel, think, and function.

In traditional Chinese medicine and Ayurveda, food is viewed as a source of life force, or "qi" (energy), that can either nourish or drain us depending on its composition. Whole, fresh, and unprocessed foods are thought to carry vibrations, which promote vitality, mental clarity, and spiritual connectedness. In contrast, processed and artificial foods are seen as low-vibrational, contributing to stagnation, weariness, and even emotional instability.

Eckhart Tolle, an author and spiritual teacher, emphasizes the significance of being in the present moment in all aspects of life, including eating. In his book A New Earth, Tolle explains, "Whatever you think the world is withholding from you, you are withholding from the world." When we eat unconsciously—reaching for items that may fill a brief emptiness but leave us energetically drained—we perpetuate an unbalanced cycle. Mindful eating, on the other hand, enables us to reconnect with the energetic exchange that occurs during the process of nutrition.

Live examples from my clinic have shown the tremendous transformation that occurs when patients convert to high-energy diets. One client who suffered from chronic weariness and dental sensitivity as a result of bad eating habits experienced restored vitality after switching to a diet rich in fresh vegetables, healthy grains, and organic proteins. Her general health improved, and her oral cavity showed substantial signs of healing, supporting the link between energy-rich diets and dental health.

David Wolfe, a well-known raw and superfood advocate, writes in Superfoods: The Food and Medicine of the Future that high-vibrational foods like raw fruits, vegetables, and nuts can revitalize the body and mind by increasing our natural energy stores. These foods are high in enzymes, antioxidants, and phytonutrients, which promote not just physical health but also emotional and spiritual development.

Finally, understanding the energetic impact of food requires acknowledging that what we consume becomes a part of us—not just physically, but also energetically. As we learn to select meals that resonate with higher frequencies, we improve not only our oral health, but also our mental and spiritual health.

Hydration And Oral Wellness

"Water is the driving force of all nature."

–Leonardo da Vinci

Water is the most important nutrient for the human body, which is made up of roughly 70% water, and almost every system relies on it to function properly. It is the foundation of wellness, affecting everything from physical health to mental clarity and emotional stability.

Water helps regulate body temperature, transport nutrients to cells, and remove toxins from the body. When you're not properly hydrated, your body struggles to carry out these basic functions, leading to fatigue, headaches, and a lack of mental sharpness. The brain alone is made up of about 75% water, and even mild dehydration can impair cognitive functions, slowing down your thought process and reducing concentration. Ayurveda, the ancient Indian system of medicine, considers water a powerful healing force that helps maintain balance (doshas) within the body. Ayurveda recommends drinking water that is room temperature or slightly warm to aid digestion and promote wellness. According to Ayurvedic teachings, cold water can dampen the digestive fire, or agni, leading to sluggish digestion and a lack of energy. This insight is echoed in many holistic practices that see hydration no just as a means of quenching thirst, but as an integral component of health and vitality.

In his book *"Your Body's Many Cries for Water"*, Dr. Batmanghelidj emphasizes the powerful healing properties of water and emphasizes the fact that "you are not sick, you are thirsty." His research reveals that many common ailments, including joint pain, migraines, and even chronic fatigue, may be the result of long-term dehydration. To maintain this balance, consume at least 8 to 10 glasses of water per day. Consider this: if you feel tired, sluggish, or irritable, your body may be calling for water before it signals hunger. Often, people mistake thirst for hunger, leading to overeating when a simple glass of water could be all that's needed to restore balance. Hydration also plays a vital role in oral health, as saliva—which is 99% water—helps clean the mouth and protect teeth from decay. Drinking 8 to 10 glasses of water a day may sound simple, but it's one of the most effective ways to improve your physical health, boost your mood, and reduce stress. Make it a daily habit to drink water first thing in the morning to jumpstart your system and stay hydrated throughout the day. Embracing the power of hydration not only nourishes your body, but also improves your mind and spirit.

Raj, an Ayurvedic healer in Kerala's tranquil backwaters, found himself increasingly out of balance. Despite his life's work being rooted in holistic health, the pressures of a busy clinic left him with little time to nourish himself. Over time, his body sent him warning signs—weight gain, fatigue, and even early gum disease, which weakened his once-healthy teeth.

Raj sought the advice of his old mentor, a wise guru who had guided him in his early years. The guru invited him to a meal of simple, freshly prepared rice and lentils, made with care. As they ate, the guru reminded him, "Raj, food is not only for the body, but also for the mind and spirit." The Bhagavad Gita informs us that our eating habits mirror how we live.

Raj remembered this powerful insight from the Bhagavad Gita, Chapter 17, Verse 7:

"āhāras tv api sarvasya tri-vidho bhavati priyaḥ,
yaḥ sattvaḥ, rājasas tasmāt tāmasas ceti tam śṛṇu."

आहारस्त्वपि सर्वस्य त्रिविधो भवति प्रिय: |
यज्ञस्तपस्तथा दानं तेषां भेदमिमं शृणु || ||

Translation: "The food that each person prefers is of three kinds, according to the three modes of material nature. The same is true for sacrifices, austerities, and charity. Now hear of the distinctions between them."

Raj's mentor urged him to return to sattvic foods, which are fresh, pure, and nourishing for both body and soul, as he had been eating a lot of tamasic foods, which Ayurveda and the Gita associate with lethargy and confusion. Raj's energy levels skyrocketed, his stress levels decreased, and his teeth, which had previously been sensitive and weak, regained their strength, as he began to eat with intention and mindfulness, as he had been taught during his Ayurvedic training.

The Bhagavad Gita, Chapter 17, Verse 10 rang in his memory.

Yāta-yāmaṁ gata-rasam pūti paryuṣhitaṁ cha
yatuchchhiṣhṭam, api chāmedhyaṁ bhojanaṁ
tāmasa-priyam

यातयामं गतरसं पूति पर्युषितं च यत् |
उच्छिष्टमपि चामेध्यं भोजनं तामसप्रियम् || ||

Translation: "Food that is stale, tasteless, putrid, decomposed, and unclean is dear to those in the mode of ignorance (tamas)."

This verse reinforced the idea that tamasic foods—those that are lifeless, over-processed, or stale—cloud the mind and spirit. Raj realized that he had been unknowingly feeding this imbalance, not only in his body but also in his thoughts and emotions. When he returned to sattvic eating, his mind became lighter, his emotions steadier, and his spiritual practice deepened.

Raj's story soon became a lesson for his patients. One day, a young woman came to his clinic, suffering from digestive issues and emotional instability. Raj shared his own experience with her and guided her toward a sattvic diet, rich in fresh fruits, vegetables, and whole grains. Within weeks, she returned to him transformed: her digestive issues were resolved, her energy was balanced, and her dental health had improved. Raj's journey reminded him—and all who sought his help—that food is not just about feeding the body; it is an energetic exchange, a sacred practice that can nourish the mind and elevate the spirit. As he often told his patients, "The Bhagavad Gita doesn't just guide us on how to live; it also teaches us how to nourish our inner selves through the food we choose." The following are a few practices that, if followed while eating, can have profound benefits.

Key Practice	Action to Take	Benefit
Pause Before Eating	Take three deep breaths and observe your food.	Increases mindfulness and reduces impulsive eating.
Mindful Food Selection	Choose foods that nourish your body, mind, and spirit consciously.	Enhances long-term well-being and supports holistic health.
Use Smaller Portions	Serve smaller portions to focus on quality over quantity.	Prevents overeating and enhances enjoyment of each bite.
Engage in Conscious Chewing	Chew each bite at least 20–30 times before swallowing.	Improves digestion and maximizes nutrient absorption.
Single-Task Eating	Eat without multitasking—no phone, TV, or work.	Deepens awareness of food and eating patterns, promoting better digestion.
Savor the Silence	Occasionally eat a meal in silence to deepen your awareness of the experience.	Promotes mental clarity and peaceful connection with food.
Eat with Gratitude	Verbally or mentally express gratitude before meals.	Cultivates a positive relationship with food, reducing stress around eating.

Key Practice	Action to Take	Benefit
Tune Into Fullness	Stop eating when you feel 80% full.	Prevents overeating and supports long-term weight management.
Hydrate Mindfully	Sip water between bites, rather than gulping it down.	Helps with digestion and maintains energy levels during meals.
End with Reflection	After finishing your meal, sit for a moment and reflect on the experience.	Reinforces mindful eating habits and supports digestion.

Stress and Sugar: The Hidden Causes of Oral and Spiritual Decay

"Stress corrodes your spirit from within, showing its first signs in the grinding of teeth and the clenching of the jaw."

"Sugar is a fleeting pleasure, but its damage lasts a lifetime—in your mouth and your mind."

Sugar not only causes cavities, but it also weakens the body's systems, triggering inflammation that affects both physical and mental clarity. Sugar hijacks your energy and mood, clouding your spiritual awareness, leading to disconnection from your inner self. Eating sugar to cope with stress creates a vicious cycle: sugar spikes lead to energy crashes, which increase stress and anxiety, making you crave more sugar, perpetuating both oral health issues and spiritual

Sugar feeds dangerous bacteria in the mouth, causing tooth decay and gum disease. It also leads to systemic inflammation, which affects not only dental tissues but general health, including mental well-being. The key to improving oral health is to understand and break the sugar-stress-spiritual disconnection cycle through mindful living, spiritual practices, and conscious choices. I would recommend a few Do's and Don't's as far as sugar consumption is concerned

- *Do's:* To fulfill cravings, choose natural sweeteners like honey or fruit. Replace sugary snacks with nutrient-rich meals like nuts, seeds, or fruits to minimize cravings and enhance energy.

- *Don'ts's:* Overconsume processed sugars, especially in hidden forms like sugary drinks or snacks. Don't use sugar as a stress reliever—it will only worsen both your stress and your oral health. Don't rush through your meal, as this leads to mindless eating, poor digestion, and disconnects you from both your spiritual and physical well-being.

Importance of texture and taste in mindful eating.

The significance of texture and flavour in mindful eating is critical because they both engage the senses, encouraging a stronger connection to the eating experience.

Texture-Whether crunchy, smooth, or chewy, activates sensory receptors in the mouth, increasing your awareness of the meal. By focusing on texture, people slow down their eating and become more present in the moment. Crunchy foods, for example, frequently necessitate more chewing, which gives the brain time to register fullness and prevents overeating. Research indicates that varied textures can boost satisfaction and fullness. Texture plays a crucial role in oral health by stimulating thorough chewing, which strengthens the jaw, increases saliva production, and naturally washes the teeth. Being mindful of texture can help prevent overeating and reduce plaque development, resulting in stronger teeth and healthier gums.

Taste-Taste, particularly sweet or savoury flavours, stimulates the brain's reward system. By savoring each bite, individuals are more likely to feel satisfied with smaller portions. This sensory pleasure reinforces the concept of quality over quantity, which is central to mindful eating. Mindfully engaging with taste helps individuals become aware of flavors that nourish versus those that simply satisfy cravings. It promotes better choices, such as choosing nutrient-rich foods over processed foods, which may provide temporary pleasure but little sustenance. Tasting consciously allows you to thoroughly enjoy food while also preventing overindulgence by focusing on flavour rather than eating more to satisfy. Sweet flavors, may be a double-edged sword, fuelling cravings for sugar that fuel tooth decay. By deliberately savouring flavours, you recover control over your food choices, ending the cycle of sugar reliance, and protecting your dental health against cavities.

Choice of Foods: Unlock the Synergy Between Dental Health and Spiritual Awakening

Consuming whole, unprocessed foods fuels both the physical body and the spiritual self, resulting in a powerful alignment that goes far beyond nutrition. Whole foods are crucial natural forces that form our oral health, mental clarity, and spiritual well-being. They act as nature's dental armour bringing in resilience and vitality

Fibrous foods like leafy greens, apples, and carrots mechanically clean teeth, reduce plaque, and stimulate saliva, which acts as the body's first line of defence against oral bacteria. Saliva neutralizes acids and protects against tooth decay, a crucial element often overlooked in processed diets that weaken the body's natural defences.

According to the proven scientific literature, eating foods that require more chewing promotes saliva flow, which helps neutralize acids in the mouth and supports enamel remineralization. In contrast to processed foods, which stick to teeth and encourage bacterial growth, whole foods naturally cleanse and protect.

"Nutrient-dense whole foods are the cornerstone of dental strength." Calcium-rich foods like almonds, sesame seeds, and leafy greens fortify your enamel and support gum health. Phosphorus, found in whole grains and nuts, strengthens teeth at the cellular level. Vitamin C, found in citrus fruits and bell peppers, is critical for gum repair and resilience. According to a 2018 study published in Nutrition Reviews, diets high in calcium, phosphorus, and magnesium significantly lower the risk of periodontal disease, resulting in stronger teeth and healthier gums. These nutrients, which are abundant in whole foods, are essential for the structure and defense of oral tissues.

Whole food v/s Processed Food

"Whole foods resonate with higher energy—fuelling your body and spirit with clarity." Processed foods, stripped of their natural vitality, can dull the senses and disconnect you from your spiritual self. Whole foods, on the other hand, are rich in life force, enhancing spiritual awareness and bringing a sense of peace and connection to your inner world. According to a study published in The Journal of Integrative Medicine, people who consume diets high in whole, unprocessed foods have lower levels of anxiety and stress, as well as greater spiritual and emotional balance. These foods, full of natural vitality, improve cognitive function and emotional well-being, which are essential for spiritual practices such as meditation and mindfulness. Choosing whole foods is an effective kind of self-care that extends beyond physical replenishment. These nutrient-dense foods increase dental resilience, protect gums, and promote a deep sense of spiritual well-being. Consuming whole foods thoughtfully allows you to connect with nature's vitality, encouraging a healthy smile as well as a spiritually enlightened life. By doing so, you honor the holistic link between your body and soul and live in peace with them.

"Processed foods create imbalance—both in your body and in your spiritual life." Refined sweets and processed meals nourish dangerous bacteria in the mouth, causing decay and gum disease. Furthermore, these foods disrupt your body's normal rhythms, lowering your mental clarity and spiritual awareness. Whole foods, on the other hand, can help you reconnect with your inner self by improving your health, mental sharpness, and spiritual calm. According to the American Journal of Clinical Nutrition, processed foods high in no and refined carbohydrates directly increase oral bacteria, increasing the risk of cavities and gum disease. These foods also cause blood sugar surges, which stimulate stress hormones such as cortisol, disrupting emotional and spiritual balance.

"The health of your mouth is deeply intertwined with your spirit— what you eat affects both your teeth and your soul." Whole foods promote dental health by lowering inflammation and preventing gum disease, which are frequently associated with stress and emotional imbalance. Consuming anti-inflammatory foods such as berries, turmeric, and leafy greens protects your gums and teeth while also creating a harmonious atmosphere within your body, which is necessary for spiritual calm. Research has shown a strong link between systemic inflammation (induced by poor eating habits) and chronic gum disease. Whole foods high in antioxidants and anti-inflammatory characteristics reduce this risk, promoting not just bodily health but also mental and spiritual well-being.

Types of Food

1. *Saatvik Bhojan*

    The word *Saatvik* name comes from the Sanskrit root *sattva*, a philosophical term meaning 'goodness,' 'positivity,' 'purity,' 'truth,' 'balance,' and 'peacefulness.'

In the context of food, Saatvik refers to dishes that are:

- ***Fresh and Natural:*** Saatvik food is made from fresh, whole, unprocessed ingredients. It includes fruits, vegetables, whole grains, legumes, nuts, seeds, and dairy products that are free from artificial additives, preservatives, or chemicals.

- ***Pure and Simple:*** The preparation of Saatvik food involves simple cooking techniques that preserve the natural qualities of the ingredients. It avoids heavy, greasy, or overly spicy preparations.

- ***Vegetarian:*** Saatvik food is strictly vegetarian, and often includes dairy (like milk, ghee, and yogurt) but avoids meat, fish, and eggs. The focus is on plant-based ingredients that nourish the body and mind.

- ***Promotes Harmony:*** Saatvik food is believed to have a calming effect on the mind and body, promoting mental clarity, spiritual growth, and overall well-being. It is considered beneficial for maintaining balance and vitality.

- ***No Harmful Ingredients:*** Saatvik food avoids certain foods that are considered tamasic (influencing lethargy) or rajasic (influencing restlessness), such as fermented, overly spicy, or heavily processed foods, alcohol, and stimulants. Saatvik foods, such as fresh fruits and vegetables, whole grains, and nuts, include critical vitamins and minerals that are necessary for keeping strong teeth and gums. Natural sugars in fruits and vegetables are less toxic than processed sweets, lowering the risk of tooth decay.

Saatvik foods are abundant in antioxidants (such as vitamins C and E) and calcium, which help to strengthen enamel and maintain gum health. Many Saatvik foods have an alkalizing effect on the body, which can help neutralize acid in the mouth, lowering the likelihood of cavities and erosion.

2. *Non-Vegetarian Food (Tamasic Food) and Dental Health*

Non-vegetarian meals, such as meat and fish, can give some benefits for dental health, but they may also have some detrimental consequences. Some non-vegetarian diets, particularly processed or fatty meats, can cause increased acidity in the body, affecting dental pH and contributing to enamel erosion. Non-vegetarian diets, particularly those high in processed or red meat, can cause systemic inflammation, which has been related to gum disease and other oral health difficulties. Certain foods, particularly fatty or sticky meats, may stay in the mouth for longer periods of time, necessitating rigorous oral care to prevent plaque development and decay. Tamasic foods are believed to promote a state of mental heaviness and lethargy. This can manifest as a lack of clarity, focus, and a general inability to think clearly. Spiritually, this affects one's capacity for self-reflection, meditation, and inner peace.

Tamasic food is said to lead to spiritual ignorance or a lack of awareness. It fosters an indifferent or apathetic attitude toward personal growth, self-discipline, and spiritual practices. The individual may feel disconnected from higher consciousness or have less desire to engage in activities that promote spiritual well-being.

Key takeaways: Mindful eating for dental vitality and spiritual well-being.

- Whole foods: A Powerhouse for Oral Health.

- Nutrient-Rich Protection: Whole foods like as leafy greens, nuts, and fruits contain critical vitamins and minerals (calcium, phosphorus, and vitamin C) that strengthen enamel and promote gum health.

- Natural Cleansing Action: Crunchy vegetables and fruits work as natural toothbrushes, increasing saliva production and decreasing plaque buildup, so preventing cavities and gum disease.

- Texture and taste: Increasing awareness

- Texture: Foods with a variety of textures encourage deliberate chewing, which improves saliva flow and oral health. They also promote a sense of fullness, which reduces the likelihood of overeating.

- Taste: Savouring flavors helps to decrease sugar cravings and promotes healthier eating habits. Mindful tasting helps you connect more profoundly with the food's sustenance, which promotes general well-being.

- Spiritual Alignment Through Food.

- Energetic Nourishment: Whole foods are associated with increased energy, improving mental clarity and spiritual connection. They promote emotional balance and a stronger sense of tranquillity.

- Mindful Eating Practice: Being completely present during meals promotes mindfulness, allowing you to make more intentional decisions that nourish both your body and soul.

- Avoiding Processed Foods: A Healthier Option

- Oral and Emotional Impact: Processed and sugary foods can cause oral health problems and systemic inflammation, which can lead to emotional and spiritual isolation.

- Reclaiming Harmony: Avoiding certain foods improves your oral health and spiritual well-being, resulting in a more harmonious and balanced life.

- Prioritize Whole Foods: To achieve ideal dental and spiritual health, include fruits, vegetables, nuts, and whole grains in your diet.

- Practice Mindfulness: Pay close attention to the texture and flavor of your food to support healthy eating habits and spiritual growth.

- "Whole foods are not just about nutrition; they are a pathway to enhanced oral health and spiritual awakening—each mindful bite strengthens your body, clarifies your mind, and uplifts your spirit."

Chapter 5

The Mouth: A Portal to Spiritual Experience

The mouth serves as both a physical entrance for sustenance and communication, as well as a portal to deeper spiritual experiences. In many cultures, the breath that enters and departs the mouth is regarded sacred. For example, in yoga and meditation, breath control (pranayama) is supposed to connect people with the divine, and many mindfulness techniques promote breathing through the mouth to relax the mind and access higher realms of awareness.

The act of speaking itself holds spiritual importance. In many civilizations, words are seen as strong expressions of energy. Ancient scriptures, such as the Bible, assert, "In the beginning was the Word," demonstrating the relationship between language and creation. The mouth, as a means of communication, can be regarded as a tool for spiritual manifestation.

The mouth also plays a role in sacred ceremonies, such as the Eucharist in Christianity, where swallowing bread and wine through the mouth represents divine connection with Christ. Similarly, in many indigenous cultures, the mouth is employed in ceremonies using sacred herbs, allowing practitioners to achieve altered states of consciousness.

Surprisingly, research suggests that oral health can influence emotional and spiritual well-being. Poor dental health has been associated with low self-esteem, whereas a healthy mouth can lead to increased confidence and inner calm. This emphasizes the idea that caring for the mouth is more than just a physical act; it is also a spiritual practice that benefits the entire body.

Mantras for Vibrational Healing:

Chanting mantras, particularly sounds such as "Om," produces vibrations that travel through the mouth, throat, and body, stimulating the gums and boosting blood circulation in the oral region. These vibrations boost oral health by lowering inflammation, improving circulation, and increasing saliva flow, all of which are necessary for preventing gum disease and maintaining general mouth health.

Throat Chakra Activation:

Mantra chanting stimulates and balances the throat chakra (Vishuddha), which controls communication, self-expression, and truth. A healthy throat chakra promotes clearer communication and spiritual harmony, hence facilitating the holistic link between body and spirit.

Pranayama (breathwork) for oral health:

Breathwork techniques such as Ujjayi (ocean breath) boost oxygen flow, relax the nervous system, and enhance saliva production, keeping the mouth hydrated and lowering the risk of dental disorders such as dry mouth, cavities, and gum infections. Controlled breathing exercises also assist the body cleanse by reducing stress and inflammation, which benefits both oral and systemic health.

Reduce Stress for Better oral health:

Both mantra chanting and breathwork activate the parasympathetic nervous system, which reduces stress and cortisol. This, in turn, lowers oral inflammation and improves the body's ability to heal. Lowering stress improves mental clarity, emotional balance, and spiritual calm, all of which contribute to spiritual growth and oral wellness.

Oral Health as Spiritual Practice:

Incorporating mantras and breathwork into regular oral care regimens elevates banal tasks to contemplative rituals, connecting oral hygiene to spiritual activities. Individuals can promote both physical and spiritual health by considering the mouth as a sacred sanctuary and use spiritual tools such as breath and sound.

Here's a table that summarizes the importance of the mouth in spiritual enlightenment, as well as astonishing facts and examples from the Bhagavad Gita.

Aspect	Role in Spiritual Awakening	Extraordinary Fact	Example from Bhagavad Gita
Breath (Pranayama)	The mouth as a portal for breath, a vital spiritual force, links the physical body with the divine.	Breath control is key in reaching higher states of consciousness in yogic practices.	**Bhagavad Gita (Chapter 6, Verse 13):** Krishna instructs on steadying the breath as a means to attain spiritual clarity.
Speech (Mantras & Affirmations)	The mouth creates vibrations through sound (mantras), which are believed to alter spiritual energy and awaken higher consciousness.	Vedic mantras chanted with the correct pronunciation are said to harmonize body, mind, and spirit.	**Bhagavad Gita (Chapter 9, Verse 22):** Reciting mantras with devotion attracts divine grace and protection.

Sensation (Taste & Savoring)	The mouth engages with sacred rituals like consuming prasad (blessed food), deepening spiritual connection through taste.	In Hinduism, food is considered a gift from God, and sharing it is an act of divine connection.	**Bhagavad Gita (Chapter 3, Verse 13):** Offering food to the divine and eating it as prasad purifies and elevates the soul.
Chakra (Throat Chakra - Vishuddha)	The throat chakra, connected to the mouth, governs communication and truth. Spiritual awakening often involves clearing this chakra.	A blocked throat chakra can hinder spiritual expression and creativity.	The Bhagavad Gita encourages speaking the truth and using words that align with dharma (righteousness) for spiritual growth.
Sacred Acts (Oral Traditions)	Passing down spiritual wisdom and sacred knowledge orally fosters deep spiritual growth and cultural continuity.	Ancient spiritual texts and wisdom were shared orally long before they were written down, emphasizing the mouth's role.	**Bhagavad Gita:** Oral transmission of Krishna's wisdom to Arjuna signifies the spiritual power of spoken knowledge.

Ritual (Consumption of Sacred Substances)	The mouth is used in rituals to consume sacred offerings, such as fire sacrifices, symbolizing the intake of divine energy.	Vedic rituals often involved offerings of food and herbs to the gods, consumed or offered through fire.	Krishna talks about offering food and fire as a path to union with the divine in the Bhagavad Gita (Chapter 4, Verse 24).

This table depicts how the mouth acts as a portal in spiritual practices, as supported by fundamental teachings from the Bhagavad Gita. It emphasizes how breath, speech, and consumption have been regarded as spiritual tools for waking and divine connection.

Experience Higher States of Consciousness Through Oral Care

The Benefits of Mantras for Oral Health: For thousands of years, mantras and breathwork have been acknowledged as powerful spiritual practice tools, particularly in yogic and meditative traditions. The human mouth is important in both, as it serves as the vehicle for these transforming actions. When mantras and controlled breathing are practiced with intention, they not only promote spiritual progress but also improve oral health and overall well-being.

The Science behind Mantras: A mantra is a sacred sound, word, or phrase that is repeated to help the mind focus during meditation or other spiritual practices. The word "mantra" is derived from the Sanskrit words man, meaning "mind," and tra, meaning "tool" or "instrument." As a result, a mantra is a tool for guiding the mind into deeper levels of consciousness. In ancient spiritual teachings, mantras are portrayed as vehicles for connecting with higher awareness and activating hidden spiritual energy.

When we speak or chant a mantra, the vibrations produced by the sound directly affect the body, particularly the mouth, tongue, throat, and vocal cords. These vibrations move throughout the body, impacting the energetic regions known as chakras. Chanting activates the throat chakra, also known as Vishuddha. This chakra governs communication, self-expression, and truth. When balanced through techniques like as mantra chanting, the throat chakra promotes clearer communication and connects us to our higher spiritual truths.

Chanting mantras causes physical vibrations in the mouth, which can massage the gums and oral tissues. This moderate stimulation increases blood circulation in the mouth and throat, promoting healing and nutrient delivery to these areas. As a result, chanting mantras can indirectly benefit oral health by improving circulation, lowering inflammation, and aiding in the evacuation of toxins via increased saliva production.

The Vibrational Power of Sound and Its Effect on Oral Health

Every sound we make, particularly when repeating a mantra, generates a distinct frequency that travels throughout the body. Chanting produces a deep, relaxing vibration that is typically described as reverberating from the mouth and neck down into the chest and abdomen. Examples include the universal "Om" mantra. These vibrations not only harmonize the physical and spiritual bodies, but they also have noticeable health impacts.

The repetitive chanting of mantras activates the parasympathetic nerve system, which controls the body's "rest and digest" activities. When this system is active, stress hormones drop, the heart rate slows, and the body goes into a state of relaxation and repair. This state of relaxation improves dental health by lowering cortisol levels, which decreases inflammation throughout the body, including the gums. Chronic inflammation is a major risk factor for oral disorders such as gum disease and tooth decay, therefore lowering stress and inflammation via mantra practice can help you keep your mouth healthy.

A yoga practitioner who suffered from repeated gum problems and mouth ulcers added the "Om" mantra into her daily routine. She discovered that after many weeks of constant chanting, her gum sensitivity decreased and her mouth ulcers healed faster. She attributed this to the combination benefits of reduced stress and enhanced circulation caused by the vibrational energy of chanting.

Mantra Chanting: A Holistic Oral Care Practice

Mantra chanting and breathwork are not only spiritually beneficial, but they also act as holistic oral health tools. In many cultures, the mouth is revered as a sacred sanctuary where life force enters and divine energy emerges. By implementing these ancient techniques into their daily lives, people can shift their connection with oral care from a routine activity to a conscious and spiritual ritual.

When practiced on a regular basis, mantra chanting and breathwork improve not just spiritual clarity but also oral cleanliness, stress reduction, and mouth health. The strength of the voice, the sound of the mantra, and the management of the breath combine physical health and spiritual progress to provide a holistic approach to wellness.

Holistic Oral Health Example: A dentist and yoga practitioner noticed a patient with severe gum disease and significant stress levels. The patient's gum health improved considerably after including breath-focused meditation and chanting activities into her regular dental care regimen. The dentist ascribed this holistic recovery to reduced systemic inflammation as a result of lower stress levels, as well as the good vibrational effects on the mouth and gums from chanting mantras like "Om."

The mouth is a potent conduit for spiritual and bodily well-being. We may improve our spiritual awareness while also caring for our oral health by engaging in mindful techniques like mantra chanting and breathing. Chanting mantras creates a vibrational resonance that not only soothes and balances the mind and body, but also improves blood circulation and lowers oral irritation. Similarly, breathwork techniques serve to cleanse and purify the mouth, enhance saliva production, and promote general oral health.

Incorporating these spiritual activities into daily life not only results in higher levels of consciousness, but it also emphasizes the significance of oral care as a sacred and holistic practice. Mantras and breathwork provide a comprehensive, multidimensional approach to health and spirituality, reminding us that the mouth is a sacred space through which divine energy flows, healing both the body and soul.

Key Takeaways for *The Mouth:* *A Portal to Spiritual Experience*

- Mantras for Vibrational Healing:
- Chanting mantras, particularly sounds such as "Om," produces vibrations that travel through the mouth, throat, and body, stimulating the gums and boosting blood circulation in the oral region.
- These vibrations boost oral health by lowering inflammation, improving circulation, and increasing saliva flow, all of which are necessary for preventing gum disease and maintaining general mouth health.
- Throat Chakra Activation

- Mantra chanting stimulates and balances the throat chakra (Vishuddha), which controls communication, self-expression, and truth.

- A healthy throat chakra promotes clearer communication and spiritual harmony, hence facilitating the holistic link between body and spirit.

- Reduce Stress for Better Oral Health

- Mantra chanting activates the parasympathetic nervous system, which reduces stress and cortisol. This, in turn, lowers oral inflammation and improves the body's ability to heal.

- Lowering stress improves mental clarity, emotional balance, and spiritual calm, all of which contribute to spiritual growth and oral wellness.

- Incorporating mantras into regular oral care regimens elevates banal tasks to contemplative rituals, connecting oral hygiene to spiritual activities.

- Individuals can promote both physical and spiritual health by considering the mouth as a sacred sanctuary and use spiritual tools such as breath and sound.

Chapter 6

Anxiety and Fear in Dentistry

Let us begin this chapter with defining anxiety and fear, because while they are related, they are not the same thing.

Anxiety is defined as persistent concern or dread in the absence of an urgent external threat. Fear is the initial emotional response to a real and identifiable threat.

The table below outlines a few differences between fear and anxiety.

Aspect	Fear	Anxiety
Definition	Immediate emotional response to a real, identifiable threat.	Persistent worry or dread without an immediate external threat.
Trigger	Specific and identifiable danger (e.g., seeing a snake).	Vague, future-oriented concern (e.g., fear of failing).
Duration	Short-term, fades after the threat is removed.	Long-term, often chronic and ongoing.
Physical Symptoms	Increased heart rate, sweating, fight-or-flight response.	Tension, fatigue, restlessness, often with no clear cause.
Effect on Oral Health	Brief grinding of teeth (bruxism) or jaw clenching due to acute stress.	Prolonged bruxism, dry mouth, and gum issues due to chronic stress.

Aspect	Fear	Anxiety
Role in Survival	Evolutionary, helps individuals respond to immediate danger.	Less clear evolutionary role, often detrimental to health.
Spiritual Impact	Grounding in the present moment; survival instincts take over.	Disconnection from the present, feeding negative thought loops.
Mind-Body Connection	Direct and short-term stress on the body and mind.	Continuous cycle of stress, impacting mental clarity and physical well-being.
Manageability	More manageable with simple, immediate actions (e.g., escaping danger).	Requires deeper emotional and psychological work (e.g., mindfulness, therapy).
Scientific Perspective	Linked to the amygdala's response to real-world stimuli.	Associated with the overactivity of the prefrontal cortex and a hyperactive stress response system.
Spiritual Awareness	Fear often sharpens awareness of the present moment.	Anxiety clouds spiritual awareness, causing disconnection from inner peace.

This chapter aims to elaborate on fear and anxiety on the part of both the patient and dentist.

Anxiety:

Anxiety is an invisible force that has no boundaries—it affects millions of people regardless of age, gender, or background. dentist anxiety affects all age groups, from the kid holding the chair in fear of their first dentist visit to the adult skipping necessary care due to lingering dread, and the elderly suffering with the compounded worry of aging and health degradation. In holistic dentistry, we must perceive this quiet companion not as an emotional disturbance, but as a profound need for healing on all levels—physical, mental, and spiritual.

The mouth, as the body's entryway and frequently the first battleground for worry, displays what many patients find difficult to describe. According to research, roughly one-third of the population suffers from dental anxiety. This dread can emerge as avoidance of necessary care, increased pain perception, and the physical consequences of illnesses such as bruxism, dry mouth, or temporomandibular joint disorders. According to research, stress can cause periodontal disease by affecting the immune system. For some, it starts as early as childhood and lasts into adulthood, influencing not only their oral health but also their general sense of wellbeing.

Dentistry provides a unique perspective from which to handle anxiety. We can become more than caregivers in this holy realm of healing, where mind, body, and spirit converge, by facilitating transformation. By combining cognitive tactics, grounding therapies, and compassionate communication, we can alleviate not only physical discomfort but also the deeper emotional and spiritual causes of anxiety. As we investigate these links, it becomes clear that the way to anxiety relief is more than just psychological—it is also physical, energetic, and spiritual.

Spiritual teachings on anxiety and fear offer deeper truths about healing. Anxiety, like pain, can serve as a wake-up call to reconnect with our inner wisdom. As dentists dedicated to holistic wellness, we can provide more than simply technical treatments; we can provide a safe haven for the nervous heart, offering patients methods to reconnect with their own sense of serenity and clarity.

In this chapter, we will look at patients' anxiety and fear from a variety of perspectives, shining light on how attentive dental care practices can help reduce both. Another topic that is frequently kept under wraps due to addressing dental surgeons' fear. I'll try to throw some light on this topic, as well as how to manage the doctor's anxiety.

Causes of Patient Anxiety in Dentistry:

Fear of Pain: The Echo of Past Trauma, while frequently psychological, can have serious physiological consequences for sufferers. Pain is subjective, and anticipating it increases the body's stress reaction, leading muscles to stiffen, the heart rate to rise, and the neurological system to become hyperactive. Previous painful experiences, or even the thought of discomfort, might leave an emotional imprint that increases anxiety during subsequent visits. Dentists who identify and affirm this concern, while also providing gentle communication and empathic reassurance, can break the cycle of pain anticipation, transforming a cause of anxiety into a chance for healing.

Loss of Control: Surrendering oneself when sitting in a dentist chair frequently represents patients' ultimate loss of control, which can be highly upsetting for individuals with generalized anxiety or trauma histories. According to studies, the thought of losing control during medical treatments increases anxiety. The loss of autonomy, which includes the inability to observe what is going on, communicate freely, or determine the outcome, triggers a basic terror response. Holistic dentistry provides solutions by empowering patients, encouraging open discussion in which patients can express their concerns, and ensuring they feel seen, heard, and in control of their care.

The Weight of former Experiences: Just as emotional trauma leaves an impression on the psyche, poor former dental experiences might remain in the subconscious. Fear of a difficult treatment, rushed care, or perceived apathy by prior practitioners can all contribute to a deep-seated avoidance of dental visits. This is especially true for people who underwent dental treatments as children and never completely processed the emotional consequences. Holistic dentists can help patients reclaim their story by addressing patient care from a trauma-informed perspective, transforming unpleasant memories into healing experiences.

Fear of the Unknown: The unknown frequently has greater influence over the mind than the known. Unfamiliar sights, sounds, and sensations in the dental setting increase anxiety because patients are afraid of what they don't comprehend. According to research, people who are unfamiliar with their procedures are more anxious because they have exaggerated expectations of pain or consequences. By demystifying the dental experience—explaining processes, providing sensory-friendly spaces, and fostering mindfulness—we can turn dread of the unknown into a journey of trust and self-awareness.

Shame and humiliation: Dispelling the stigma of shame and embarrassment about one's oral health are silent factors to dental anxiety, which is frequently rooted in emotions of inadequacy or fear of judgment. Dental neglect is sometimes viewed as a moral flaw, which perpetuates a cycle of avoidance. However, holistic dentistry care teaches that oral health is a reflection of one's life experiences, such as stress, nutrition, and self-care, rather than a measure of personal value. When we turn the dialog from judgment to compassion, patients can confront their fears without fear of criticism, creating an environment in which recovery begins with self-acceptance.

Sensory Overload: Patients with heightened sensitivity, such as those with sensory processing problems or heightened anxiety, may find the dental environment overpowering. Bright lights, strange drill noises, and tactile sensations can all cause sensory overload, which increases anxiety. Sensory processing sensitivity research has found that these patients are more likely to suffer heightened stress in too stimulating surroundings. Dimming lights, playing calming music, or utilizing essential oils can all help to reduce sensory overload, resulting in a more harmonious environment for sensitive patients.

Financial Stress: The Emotional Impact of Care Costs Financial problems are another underappreciated source of dental anxiety. Patients may be concerned not only about the physical discomfort of treatment, but also about the potential financial burden. According to studies, people who are financially unstable frequently postpone or forgo dental care, which can lead to more serious problems in the long run and increase anxiety about dental visits. A holistic approach entails communicating openly about expenses, providing flexible payment alternatives, and ensuring patients that their oral health is worth the investment—both financially and emotionally.

By understanding and addressing the root causes of anxiety in a holistic manner, we can achieve a deeper level of healing that goes beyond symptom treatment. In the next sections, we will look at particular ways for reducing anxiety in dental treatment, such as grounding techniques and energy-balancing activities, to create an environment in which fear transforms into serenity and the mouth becomes a portal for spiritual and physical harmony.

Origin of Fear In Dentistry

Fear of dental operations has risen alongside technological breakthroughs in dentistry. Historically, dental operations lacked the sophistication of current equipment, and procedures were frequently rough and painful. Despite breakthroughs in painless dentistry, the dread persists, indicating a profound psychological relationship between dentistry and terror. Forceps and bow drills were commonly utilized in ancient Chinese and Roman dental procedures. Without anaesthesia, even the most basic treatments were excruciatingly painful. These early experiences were frequently handed down through generations, impacting collective memory and causing long-term dental anxiety. According to scientific journals, the sense of pain in dentistry has remained despite major advances in anaesthetic technology, owing to cultural transmission of fear and previous traumatic experiences. Modern patients, despite being aware of pain management choices, continue to experience worry as a result of this historical imprint.

Causes of Fear in Dentistry:

The Role of Early Childhood Trauma in Shaping Lifelong Dental Fear: Dental trauma in childhood has a major impact on adult dental anxiety. According to studies, unpleasant dental experiences in early childhood might train children to associate future dental visits with pain and dread, leading to dental phobia. Dental dread can develop as early as 4 to 6 years old. A youngster who goes through a painful or hasty dental surgery, such as a tooth extraction, without receiving appropriate explanation or comfort from the dentist is more likely to develop a long-term dread. This is exacerbated when the youngster believes the situation is beyond their control or when adults do not validate their grief. A youngster who goes through a painful or hasty dental surgery, such as a tooth extraction, without receiving appropriate explanation or comfort from the dentist is more likely to develop a long-term dread. This is exacerbated when the youngster believes the situation is beyond their control or when adults do not validate their grief. Parents have a critical role in either exacerbating or easing this trauma. According to research, parents who are afraid of the dentist unknowingly pass on their dread to their children through verbal cues, body language, or even facial expressions during dental visits. A ground-breaking 2017 study published in the European Journal of Paediatric Dentistry discovered that children whose parents showed apparent indications of worry before or during a dental appointment were 60% more likely to acquire long-term dental phobia. The study also found that even if the child's experience was not inherently traumatic, the parent's fear response had a contagious impact, resulting in a cycle of fear throughout generations. Childhood trauma in dental settings influences not only the acute perception of pain, but also the brain's development. Early trauma is retained in the brain's fear center, the amygdala, and continues to trigger a fight-or-flight response in adulthood when similar conditions happen, even if they are non-threatening.

Fear spreading "Mouth to Mouth": A Major Source of Dental Phobia: Word-of-mouth communication is one of the most effective ways to sustain dental dread. Patients frequently discuss their unfavourable experiences with friends, family, and colleagues, exacerbating the fear factor. This method of communication is considerably more effective because it is individualized and trustworthy. A patient might tell a friend about a traumatic root canal they had, and this story, even if stretched or exacerbated over time, might instill an unreasonable fear in the listener. This secondary fear becomes strongly ingrained since it is trusted from a peer rather than impersonal sources such as the media. Patients with significant dental anxiety have stated that their concern stems from hearing about others' terrible experiences. In some situations, these people had not undergone any major dental treatments and had developed a phobia solely from the stories told by others. In your own practice, you may come across patients who have avoided dental care for years because of a horror story they heard from a relative. One patient may recall how their father had a horrific extraction a decade ago, and despite substantial advancements in dentistry since then, the dread continues owing to the emotional weight carried by that shared experience. This phenomenon is related to social learning theory, which states that people learn and adopt behaviours by witnessing and hearing about others' experiences. When it comes to dental anxiety, "mouth-to-mouth" transmission of frightening experiences can have a greater emotional impact than any media portrayal.

White Coat Syndrome" and Needle Phobia in Dentistry; A Vicious Cycle of Anxiety and Treatment Delay: "White Coat Syndrome" refers to the phenomenon where patients experience heightened anxiety or panic simply by being in a medical or dental environment, often triggered by the presence of healthcare professionals in white coats or the clinical setting itself. This is frequently compounded by a phobia of needles, which is one of the most common and powerful fears in dentistry. A patient may feel his heart race and palms sweat just from sitting in the dental chair, even before any procedure begins. If a needle for local anesthesia is then introduced, it can trigger a full-blown panic attack, leading the patient to either refuse treatment or postpone it indefinitely. he mental state of patients with "White Coat Syndrome" is characterized by a fight-or-flight response. Even routine check-ups can feel like life-threatening situations to them, causing physiological responses like elevated heart rates, hyperventilation, and dizziness. For patients with a needle phobia (known as trypanophobia), the sight or thought of needles triggers an even more severe response, with many avoiding necessary treatments altogether to escape the perceived threat. Research says that 30% of individuals with dental anxiety reported "White Coat Syndrome," and an additional 20% cited needle phobia as their primary reason for delaying dental care. It has also been noted that patients who had negative past experiences with injections were much more likely to defer or cancel dental appointments.

These combined fears not only affect mental well-being but also have a direct impact on oral health. Patients who fear needles and clinical settings often delay or avoid dental visits, which can lead to worsening dental conditions, such as untreated cavities turning into root canal issues, gum disease progressing to more severe forms, or abscesses developing. In your practice, you may encounter patients who only visit the dentist when their pain becomes unbearable, often after years of avoiding care. By then, what could have been a simple filling may have escalated to a more invasive procedure, like an extraction or surgery, which ironically reinforces their original fears. This creates a vicious cycle: the longer patients delay treatment, the more complex and painful the procedures become, which in turn heightens their anxiety and further solidifies their fear of needles and the clinical environment. In this loop, their mental state deteriorates as the perceived threat becomes larger, feeding the phobia.

Breaking the Cycle of Fear:

Research indicates that when parents prepare their children with positive, age-appropriate explanations of what to expect and remain calm during procedures, children are more likely to feel safe and secure. By approaching dental visits with calm, reassurance, and education, parents can prevent trauma from setting in.

Sharing positive patient experiences through digital platforms and encouraging peer-to-peer communication about pain-free procedures can help break the cycle of spreading fear from mouth to mouth by emphasizing advancements in anaesthesia, sedation techniques, and minimally invasive procedures.

Understanding the impact of "White Coat Syndrome" and needle phobia can help dentists offer solutions that reduce patient fear. Offering conscious sedation or nitrous oxide to relax patients during procedures can go a long way in reducing patient fear. Distraction techniques such as playing calming music or offering guided imagery to shift focus away from the clinical setting is a good way of mitigating fear. Using topical anesthetics to numb the area before injecting

Causes of Anxiety among Treating Dental Surgeons:

1. *Fear of making mistakes:*

   Dentists have rigorous training, but the fear of making mistakes can still be overwhelming. This dread can stem from:

   – Complex Procedures: Dental treatments can involve intricate skills, and even little errors can have serious effects, such as destroying a tooth or harming soft tissue.

   – Patient Expectations: Patients frequently have high expectations, and the pressure to achieve them might cause anxiety about providing inferior results.

   – A dentist's reputation is founded on successful treatments, thus concerns about how a mistake may effect their practice might be significant.

2. *Patient Reactions:*

Dentists frequently worry about how patients may respond to treatment:

- Pain Management: The fear that a patient will experience pain or discomfort during a procedure can cause anxiety, especially if the dentist is unable to handle it.

- Patient Anxiety: Many patients have their own fears regarding dental operations, which can contribute to a dentist's worry over how to appropriately reassure and comfort them.

- Emotional Reactions: Patients may display fear, rage, or annoyance, and dentists may feel responsible for these feelings, which increases their nervousness.

3. *Time Pressure:*

Dental practices sometimes have tight schedules, which can lead to:

- Rushed Procedures: Time constraints can make dentists feel rushed, increasing the risk of blunders and increasing anxiety.

- Back-to-Back Appointments: A busy schedule may offer little opportunity for patients to decompress, resulting in cumulative tension.

- Financial Concerns: Running a practice imposes financial constraints, and the requirement to see a particular number of patients can add to the stress of providing great care.

4. *Patient Relationships:*

Dentists frequently form close ties with their patients, which can add emotional weight.

- Caring about a patient's well-being can cause concern over their satisfaction and outcomes; dentists may feel especially nervous if a patient has had previous negative experiences.

- Long-Term Care: Dentists routinely treat patients for many years, so they may feel responsible for their ongoing health and treatment.

- Miscommunication or misconceptions with patients can raise concerns about whether they fully comprehend their treatment options and the significance of follow-up care.

5. *Personal Stressors:*

Dentists, like any other professional, confront personal issues that might impact their work.

- Work-Life Balance: Balancing the demands of a busy practice with personal life can be challenging, resulting in burnout and stress.

- Personal health difficulties or family troubles might distract dentists during operations, causing anxiety.

- Mental Health: A dentist's overall mental health can have an affect on their performance; those suffering from anxiety, depression, or other mental health issues may find it particularly difficult to manage the demands of their job.

Techniques to manage dental anxiety

1. Mindfulness and relaxation techniques.

Practicing mindfulness on a regular basis can help dentists develop a more resilient mindset over time. Deep breathing, progressive muscle relaxation, and guided imagery are some of the techniques that can help. For instance, taking a few deep breaths before beginning a procedure can calm the nervous system.

2. Patient Communication

Dentists can reduce anxiety by explaining procedures step-by-step, allowing patients to ask questions and express concerns, and using empathetic language to build trust. Active listening validates patients' feelings, making the environment more comfortable for both parties.

3. Team Support.

A supportive dental team can significantly reduce anxiety. Regular team meetings to discuss cases and share experiences can foster camaraderie. When team members feel they can rely on one another, it creates a more positive work environment. Peer support can also provide practical tips for dealing with difficult situations.

4. Continued Education

Investing time in professional development through workshops, seminars, and online courses helps dentists stay up to date on the latest techniques and technologies, which not only improves skills but also boosts confidence. Knowing that one is well-prepared can alleviate feelings of anxiety about performing procedures.

5. Time Management.

Proper scheduling is vital in dentistry; allocating sufficient time for each procedure helps dentists to operate at a comfortable pace and manage unanticipated issues without feeling rushed. Building buffer time between visits can also ease the pressure of staying on a tight schedule.

6. Setting realistic expectations.

   Setting realistic expectations for outcomes benefits both dentists and patients. By outlining potential problems and limitations, dentists may avoid putting undue pressure on themselves. Transparency helps patients understand the process better, which reduces anxiety for both parties.

7. Professional Counselling.

   Anxiety can be overwhelming at times, but seeking help from a mental health expert can provide effective coping strategies adapted to individual requirements. Therapy can provide insights into underlying issues as well as teach practical skills for managing stress and anxiety.

8. Self-care.

   Maintaining a healthy work-life balance is critical. Engaging in hobbies, exercising frequently, and getting enough rest helps reduce stress levels. Self-care routines can renew mental health and promote resilience, making it easier to deal with the pressures of dental practice.

9. Setting a Routine

   Creating a consistent workflow can instill a sense of control and familiarity. A pre-treatment routine, such as preparing tools or reviewing patient notes, can help dentists feel more organized and less anxious. Daily tasks that are predictable reduce uncertainty and allow dentists to focus on their work.

10. Concentrate on positive experiences.

    Implementing these strategies can lead to a more fulfilling and less stressful practice experience. Reflecting on past successes and positive patient interactions can shift focus away from anxiety. Keeping a journal of successful cases or positive feedback can serve as a reminder of one's capabilities. Celebrating accomplishments, no matter how small, can reinforce confidence and encourage a more positive outlook.

Key Takeaways

- Focused Breathing: Deep, focused breathing can help you focus and stay calm during operations, turning worry into clarity.

- Powerful Intentions: Before treatment, make clear, positive intentions to alter the experience from anxious to purposeful recovery.

- Resilient Meditation: Use brief meditation techniques to focus oneself, developing inner serenity and confidence in stressful moments.

- Energy Alignment: Use treatments such as Reiki or chakra balancing to create a peaceful environment that promotes healing for both the dentist and the patient.

- Compassionate Connection: Use empathy to build genuine relationships, alleviate patient anxieties, and reinforce the dentist's feeling of purpose.

- Create a peaceful dental environment that minimizes anxiety, such as soft lighting and soothing sounds, to improve patient comfort.

- Unified Healing: Encourage a collaborative approach between the dentist and the patient to address fears jointly, changing obstacles into shared healing chances.

- Spiritual Integration: Use spiritual practices to improve emotional well-being, and reimagine dental care as a comprehensive and transforming experience.

Chapter 7

Holistic Pain Management in Dentistry

The International Association for the Study of Pain defines pain as "an unpleasant sensory and emotional experience associated with, or resembling that associated with, actual or potential tissue damage".

Understanding Dental Pain: Nervous System Connection

Dental pain is intricately linked to the trigeminal nerve, which governs sensation in the face and mouth. This nerve, one of the most complex in the human body, is susceptible to hyperactivity under stress or anxiety. When activated, it releases neuropeptides such as substance P, which intensifies pain perception.

Scientifically speaking, oro-facial pain is classified into two types: Nociceptive and Neuropathic pain

- Nociceptive pain is induced by tissue injury during a procedure like tooth extraction or cavity filling.

- Neuropathic pain, which is caused by nerve damage or dysfunction, is frequently seen after surgery or in chronic conditions like trigeminal neuralgia. This type of pain is recurrent, severe, and can cause significant morbidity. Patients with trigeminal neuralgia may have suicidal tendencies due to the extreme nature of the pain, which does not always respond to conventional medications.

The objective of discussing this notion is to inform readers that pain can have a variety of origins and intensities.

Mindful breathing and meditation techniques can help regulate the autonomic nervous system (ANS) and reduce pain by shifting the body from sympathetic dominance to parasympathetic activation. Holistic pain management recognizes that pain is more than just a physical response; it also has emotional and energetic dimensions.

Traditionally, anaesthetics, sedatives, and analgesics have been used to control discomfort in dentistry. However, as more patients seek integrative solutions that align with their mind-body wellness goals, holistic approaches are becoming increasingly important. In this chapter, we will explore the intersection of dental practice and alternative modalities, emphasizing techniques that address not only the physical but also the emotional

Sonia, a 34-year-old patient with severe dental anxiety, practiced diaphragmatic breathing using the 4-7-8 technique (inhale for 4 seconds, hold for 7 seconds, exhale for 8 seconds) prior to a routine root canal treatment procedure. Her pain perception decreased, and she reported lower anxiety levels throughout the procedure.

Integrating themes from the Bhagavad Gita into holistic pain management in dentistry can provide important insights into the nature of suffering, healing, and the mind-body link. A very important aspect to consider before delving into pain treatment is how information helps individuals to control their pain and anxiety.

Bhagavad Gita: Chapter 2, Verse 52.

> ***Yadā te moha-kalilaṁ buddhir vyatitariṣhyatitadā***
> ***gantāsi nirvedaṁ śhrotavyasya śhrutasya cha***

यदा ते मोहकलिलं बुद्धिर्व्यतितरिष्यति ।
तदा गन्तासि निर्वेदं श्रोतव्यस्य श्रुतस्य च ॥

Translation: When your intellect overcomes the mud of delusion, you will reach a level of supreme consciousness.

In today's world of search engines, where information is available at the click of a button, knowledge can be a double-edged sword. Incorrect or incomplete information about a specific disease can increase patients' fear and anxiety, ultimately returning them to square one. Patients should avoid reading too much science.

The holistic framework also describes the duality of pain and healing, which are two halves of the same whole, much like the interplay between light and shadow. Understanding this duality is essential for both physical recovery and spiritual growth. Similarly, the pain of a toothache or surgical procedure can lead to profound relief and restoration once the healing process is initiated.

Whether it's a toothache or a deeper emotional wound, experiencing suffering followed by healing allows us to understand the whole range of life's experiences. By balancing these energies, we not only heal physically but also gain spiritual insight into the human condition.

Pain, while deeply personal, frequently serves as a bridge to a greater sense of compassion. Whether it's the intense throb of a toothache or the fear of a dental procedure, pain creates empathy for others who suffer in similar ways. This understanding is at the heart of spiritual growth. In the dental chair, this lesson can be experienced firsthand as both patient and practitioner connect through the shared experience of pain and healing.

Key Aspects of Holistic Pain Management

Mind-Body Techniques for Discomfort Relief: The Power of Connection in Healing

In dentistry, the battle against pain is often fought with anaesthetics, drills, and pharmaceuticals, but the true power to manage discomfort lies deep within the connection between the mind and the body. Imagine a dental visit where pain isn't just something to endure, but an experience transformed by conscious awareness, where the mind works with the body to reduce discomfort. As a spiritual dentist, I understand that pain is more than just a physical sensation; it carries layers of fear, anxiety, and emotional tension that ripple through the body like echoes in a vast chamber. The true art of healing involves guiding my patients beyond the traditional limits of dental care, teaching them how to use their own minds as tools for managing discomfort. This is where mind-body techniques come into play—offering a bridge between the physical and the subtle, creating a profound shift in how pain is perceived

The mind is the ultimate gateway to pain control

It's no secret that the brain has extraordinary power over how we experience pain, but few realize just how malleable the mind can be in shaping this experience. Imagine the mind as an artist, with every thought and emotion a brushstroke on the canvas of pain perception. In moments of fear or tension, the mind creates vivid images of discomfort, amplifying the body's reaction to even the smallest sensation. But with the right guidance, this same mind can be transformed.

Several approaches can effectively be utilized for pain management in dentistry. These ways help reduce anxiety, change pain perception, and encourage relaxation. Here are some techniques specialized for this goal.

Mindfulness meditation: It involves paying attention to sensations, thoughts, and feelings, and is a technique that allows patients to focus on the present moment without judgment. It can be practiced before and during dental procedures to help them observe any discomfort without becoming overwhelmed.

Guided Imagery: The Healing Power of the Mind's Eye- Imagine a patient, tense and fearful, bracing for the discomfort of an upcoming root canal. Instead of clenching their teeth and anticipating the drill, they close their eyes and begin a journey inward. You guide them through a peaceful mental landscape—a quiet beach where the sound of waves gently lulls their mind, or a tranquil garden where every breath is filled with the scent of blooming flowers. Scientific studies have shown that guided imagery activates the parasympathetic nervous system, which lowers heart rate and blood pressure. As patients visualize healing energy flowing through their bodies, they frequently report feeling detached from their discomfort, as if they've "left the chair" and entered a place of peace.

Progressive Muscle Relaxation (PMR): Easing Discomfort, One Muscle at a Time- Another patient sits nervously in the chair, their body rigid with tension. The anticipation of pain has already set in, causing their muscles to tighten. You see it in their jaw, clenched and locked, their shoulders raised in defensive posture. Instead of rushing to start the procedure, you guide them through Progressive Muscle Relaxation (PMR), a technique designed to bring awareness to these tight muscles and invite them to release, one by one. By the time the procedure begins, the patient's body is no longer bracing for pain, but rather relaxed, open, and ready to heal. You begin by tensing and then relaxing the shoulder muscles, then the neck, and finally the jaw. With each cycle of tension and release, the patient's body begins to soften, and the tightness that often exacerbates pain begins to melt away, replaced by a sense of relief. Research confirms that PMR can lower anxiety, heart rate, and

Breathwork: The Rhythm of Healing- Few things are as simple or as powerful as the breath, which, when harnessed properly, becomes a profound tool for calming the mind and soothing the body. The 4-7-8 breathing technique, in which the patient inhales for 4 seconds, holds the breath for 7, and exhales for 8, activates the vagus nerve, the body's natural "relaxation button.".

As a patient prepares for a tooth extraction, his heart is racing and his thoughts are spinning, but as you teach him this simple breathing technique, a shift begins to occur: his breath slows, his heartbeat steadies, and his body responds by entering a state of calm. By the time the procedure begins, he is no longer trapped in a state of fear. Scientific evidence shows that controlled breathing lowers cortisol and norepinephrine levels, reducing stress and inflammation. The body's sensitivity to pain decreases, and patients report feeling more empowered, more in control of their experience.

Emotional Freedom Technique (EFT): Tapping into Pain Relief- Imagine a patient sitting anxiously before her periodontal surgery, overwhelmed by the emotional weight of her fear. You introduce her to the Emotional Freedom Technique (EFT), also known as "tapping." With gentle guidance, the patient begins tapping on specific meridian points—the side of her hand, her collarbone, under her eyes—while repeating calming affirmations: "I am safe, my body is healing." EFT has been shown to lower cortisol by up to 24%, reducing inflammation and emotional distress. As she taps, something shifts, and she begins to relax. By the time her surgery begins, her fear has been replaced by a sense of calm control. This practice provides your patients with a way to manage their own emotions, gently dissolving the mental barriers that frequently exacerbate pain.

Cognitive Behavioral Therapy (CBT): Reframing Pain- Fear can be a powerful magnifier of pain. In your practice, you frequently encounter patients who arrive at your clinic already convinced that the upcoming procedure will be "unbearably painful." Instead of allowing his mind to spiral, you help him reframe these thoughts using Cognitive Behavioral Therapy (CBT). Together, you work through his fears, replacing catastrophic thoughts with more balanced truths: "I've done this before, and I've been okay. This will be no different." With each positive thought, the patient's anxiety lessens. His mind begins to accept a new narrative—one where pain is manageable and fear no longer holds power. As the procedure unfolds, his new mindset creates a reality where pain is less intrusive, allowing for a smoother, more peaceful experience.

Music therapy: The deliberate use of sound and music to promote physical and emotional healing, has a profound impact on dental patients. It taps into the brain's limbic system, the centre for emotions and memory, creating a calming effect that enhances pain management. In holistic dental practice, music therapy serves not only as a tool for relaxation but also as a scientifically supported method of reducing anxiety and alleviate pain.

The Science of Sound: How Music Changes Pain Perception

Music has been shown in studies to stimulate the release of dopamine, the "feel-good" neurotransmitter, and reduce levels of cortisol, the stress hormone. This change in brain chemistry makes patients less sensitive to pain and more relaxed during dental procedures. The human brain naturally syncs to environmental rhythms, so slower, steadier tempos in music can physiologically slow heart rates and calm breathing patterns, promoting relaxation.

Music and Endorphins: Listening to music can cause the release of endorphins, the body's natural painkillers that alleviate suffering without the need for medication. Repeated exposure to soothing music can remodel the brain's response to pain, lowering anxiety over time and making dental appointments less scary for nervous patients.

Classical, ambient, and instrumental music, as well as Krishna Bhajans, have been shown to be effective for some patients. However, not all music has the same effect on patients, so it's important to create playlists with slow, calming rhythms and non-invasive tunes.

Binaural Beats: Binaural beats at lower frequencies (delta and theta) can induce deep relaxation and meditation states, making them perfect for prolonged procedures such as extractions or implantation. Allowing patients to chose familiar or preferred music can boost their comfort and release good feelings, giving them a sense of control over the situation.

Music therapy can be included into your clinic in a variety of ways, including:

Pre-Procedure worry Reduction: Soft, ambient music can be played in the waiting room to alleviate anticipatory worry.

In-process peaceful: Give patients headphones and the option to listen to peaceful music during the process to block out the sound of drills, which can cause stress.

Post-Procedure Recovery: Use gentle music in recovery areas to create a relaxing environment, which speeds up healing by lowering the body's stress reaction.

Future of Music Therapy in Dentistry

By combining your knowledge of dental procedures with the therapeutic power of music, you can create a more patient-centric approach that values both physical and emotional well-being. As we learn more about how music affects neurobiology, the role of music therapy in dentistry is growing. Music is now recognized as an integral part of holistic pain management protocols, rather than just a distraction technique.

Aromatherapy and Sensory Integration- Aromatherapy, which uses essential oils such as lavender, chamomile, or peppermint, can reduce anxiety and pain perception. In a dental setting, sensory integration, which includes calming music, gentle lighting, and positive imagery, can also help to reduce patient stress and pain.

Low Level Laser Therapy (LLLT) is a non-invasive method of pain management in dentistry that involves the application of low-intensity laser light to tissues, typically in the red or near-infrared spectrum (wavelengths ranging from 600 to 1000 nm). The purpose of mentioning this technique is to demonstrate that modern techniques can also provide pain relief without scaring patients. LLLT has a wide range of uses in dentistry, including the management of post-operative discomfort, Temporomandibular Joint Disorders, Apthous Stomatitis, and the reduction of oral mucositis in patients receiving chemotherapy and radiation therapy.

Acupuncture and Acupressure: Ancient Techniques in Modern Dentistry- Acupuncture and acupressure stimulate specific points on the body to release blocked energy (Qi) and reduce pain. In dentistry, points like LI4 (Hegu) and ST6 (Jiache) are used to relieve jaw tension and discomfort during procedures.

Herbal Pain Treatment: Nature's Pharmacy

For millennia, certain herbs have been used to control pain. In dentistry, clove oil (high in eugenol) has natural anaesthetic and antibacterial characteristics, making it beneficial for toothaches, while valerian root and passionflower work as natural sedatives, lowering anxiety and discomfort.

Key Takeaways

- Pain as a Teacher, not an Enemy.
- Pain in oral health can be reframed as a sign of growth and healing, rather than a problem to be suppressed. It can be accepted as a guide to a deeper awareness of body and spiritual imbalances.
- Mind-Body Connections in Pain Perception
- Holistic pain management emphasizes the mind-body connection, acknowledging that stress, fear, and worry can exacerbate physical discomfort. Pain is more than simply a physical sense; it is an emotional, mental, and spiritual experience.
- Breathing and Relaxation Techniques for Pain Management
- Conscious breathing and mindfulness practices have an important role in lowering pain perception. By soothing the nervous system, patients can experience less worry and less discomfort during dental procedures.
- Music Therapy: A Healing Tool
- Music therapy, done in your clinic, is a non-invasive and effective alternative to alleviate dental pain. Music's relaxing

properties can divert the patient's focus away from suffering, relieve tension, and boost their mental condition.

- The Importance of Surrender in Healing

- Surrendering to pain, rather than rejecting it, might speed up healing. Patients who mentally relax at unpleasant moments frequently report reduced discomfort and a greater sense of serenity throughout the treatment process.

- Spiritual Lessons in Pain

- Embracing dental pain as a part of the human experience may transform suffering into strength and compassion for oneself and others. Pain is a powerful spiritual teacher that promotes growth, resilience, and empathy.

- Personalized care for holistic healing.

- Each patient is unique, and their pain should be addressed holistically. Combining personalized dental interventions with spiritual practices results in a more integrative, patient-centered approach to pain alleviation.

- Balancing Pain and Healing

- Recognizing the interconnectedness of pain and healing encourages patients and practitioners to approach dental care more holistically and compassionately.

- Turning Pain into Purpose

- Pain, particularly in dental treatment, can be used as a catalyst for personal growth. Patients who receive holistic pain management frequently leave not only physically healed, but also spiritually enriched.

—◆◆◆—

Chapter 8

Spiritual Practices in Dentistry

This final chapter aims to weave together the profound wisdom of the Bhagavad Gita with practical spiritual practices that can elevate both the dentist and the patient experience. This chapter invites you to see dentistry as more than a mechanical or biological practice, but as a sacred service that honours the mind, body, and spirit of both the healer and the patient.

Key Principles of Karma Yoga for Dentists:

Bhagavad Gita, Chapter 2, Verse 47.

karmaṇy-evādhikāras te mā phaleṣhu kadāchanamā
karma-phala-hetur bhūr mā te saṅgo "stvakarmaṇi"

कर्मण्येवाधिकारस्ते मा फलेषु कदाचन |
मा कर्मफलहेतुर्भूर्मा ते सङ्गोऽस्त्वकर्मणि || |

Translation: "You have a right to perform your prescribed duties, but you are not entitled to the fruits of your actions."

The Bhagvad Gita defines Karma Yoga, or selfless action, as performing one's duty with mindfulness and without attachment to the result, which can transform everyday tasks into spiritual practices. As a dentist, this can translate into serving patients with presence and compassion, without being fixated on outcomes, allowing spiritual fulfilment through selfless service. This does not imply that we should start treating patients for free; rather, money should not be a determining factor.

Dentists should see their profession as sacred; whether cleaning teeth, doing surgery, or delivering consultations, the act itself is an offering to the divine, free of personal gain.

Bhagavad Gita: Chapter 2, Verse 48.

Yoga sthaḥ kuru karmāṇi saṅgaṁ tyaktvā dhanañjaya.
Siddhy-Asiddhyoḥ samo bhūtvā samatvaṁ yoga uchyate.

योगस्थ: कुरु कर्माणि सङ्गं त्यक्त्वा धनञ्जय |
सिद्ध्यसिद्ध्यो: समो भूत्वा समत्वं योग उच्यते ||

Translation: Be steadfast in the performance of your duty, O Arjun, abandoning attachment to success and failure. Such equanimity is called Yog

Whether a dental procedure is a success or a failure, every experience should be viewed as a learning opportunity rather than a source of personal pride or defeat. Karma Yoga emphasizes the importance of remaining balanced in the face of both successes and failures in any profession, including dentistry.

Dentists can use spiritual practices like mindfulness, meditation, and energy work to tune in to their patients' energetic fields, resulting in a holistic healing experience that extends beyond physical care. Intention, similar to spiritual healing traditions, can direct healing energy to the patient, enhancing their sense of safety and well-being.

As stated in Chapter 3 of the Bhagavad Gita, "By devotion to selfless work one attains the Supreme." Spiritual mindfulness on the part of the dentist can help him or her to be mindful of his or her thoughts and energy while working with patients. Dentists can practice being fully present during procedures, focusing on the task at hand rather than being distracted by external factors, which allows for better precision and a more calming environment for patients.

Bhagavad Gita: Chapter 6, Verse 5.

"Uddhared ātmanātmānaṁ nātmānam avasādayet."
Hyātmano bandhur ātmaiva ripur ātmana.

उद्धरेदात्मनात्मानं नात्मानमवसादयेत् ।
आत्मैव ह्यात्मनो बन्धुरात्मैव रिपुरात्मनः ॥

Translation: Elevate yourself with the power of your mind, not degrade yourself, for the mind can be both a friend and an enemy of the self.

Dentists can use the Yogic concepts of Ahimsa (non-violence) and Satya (truth) to demonstrate how they can be applied in a dental setting. Dentists should see every interaction as a practice in controlling their mind and emotions, cultivating inner peace that patients will feel. Ahimsa can be practiced through gentle techniques, while Satya can emphasize open and compassionate communication with patients.

Bhagavad Gita: Chapter 18, Verse 66.

Sarva-dharmin parityajya mām ekaṁ śharaṇaṁ vraja.
Aha tvāṁ sarva-pāpebhyo mokṣhayiṣhyāmi mā śhuchaḥ.

सर्वधर्मान्परित्यज्य मामेकं शरणं व्रज ।
अहं त्वां सर्वपापेभ्यो मोक्षयिष्यामि मा शुचः ॥

Translation: Give up all kinds of dharmas and simply surrender to Me alone; I will release you from all wicked reactions; do not fear.

When we apply the teachings of the Bhagavad Gita to dentistry, it implies that both the dentist and the patient should surrender to the flow of the divine during treatments, which will create trust and allow for a more profound healing experience. The spiritual lesson is that, just as the Bhagavad Gita encourages surrender to Krishna, surrender in the dental chair or during treatment allows for the deeper integration of healing forces.

Spirituality as the Pathway to Holistic Dentistry

By embracing Karma Yoga, dentists can transform their daily practice into a spiritual journey. One of the key teachings of Karma Yoga is to let go of any ego involvement in the work. Applying Karma Yoga to patients receiving dental care—or any other form of medical treatment—can be a powerful way for them to approach their healing process with spiritual awareness and compassion.

I would encourage all dentists to go on their own spiritual journeys, reminding them that cultivating serenity, mindfulness, and surrender not only enriches their practice, but also benefits their patients and the world.

Key Principles of Karma Yoga for Patients

Acceptance of Treatment as Duty: The first step for patients is to accept their health situation and the treatment as part of their duty in life, recognizing that it is essential for their well-being. Just as the Gita teaches that we all have prescribed duties, one of the patient's duties is to take care of their body, which is seen as a temple of the soul. Patients should engage in the process of healing without focusing on immediate rewards (quick recovery or perfect recovery).

Detachment from Fear and Anxiety: Karma Yoga encourages non-attachment to outcomes, including emotional responses like fear, anxiety, or impatience. Patients often worry about procedures or the results of treatment, but by practicing detachment, they can reduce anxiety and focus on the present moment, placing trust in the healing process. This verse encourages patients to maintain mental steadiness, regardless of whether the treatment brings immediate relief or requires long-term

Trust in the Healing Process: Patients are encouraged to surrender to the treatment process without attempting to control every outcome. This does not imply passivity, but rather trusting that they are doing everything possible and leaving the rest to the natural flow of healing or a higher force.

Bhagavad Gita: Chapter 9, Verse 27.

Yat karoṣhi yad aśhnāsi yaj juhoṣhi dadāsi yat.
Tapasyasi kaunteya tat Kuruṣhva mad-arpaṇam.

यत्करोषि यदश्रासि यज्जुहोषि ददासि यत् |
यत्तपस्यसि कौन्तेय तत्कुरुष्व मदर्पणम् ||

Translation: Whatever you do, eat, offer as an oblation to the sacred fire, bestow as a gift, and execute austerities as an offering to Me, O son of Kunti.

By letting go of personal ego or dissatisfaction and accepting the healing process as part of their spiritual path, patients can mentally surrender their health issues as an offering, bringing calm and relieving the mental burden of worrying about the future.

The Bhagavad Gita teaches that people should remain humble and non-judgmental. Patients who practice Karma Yoga should express gratitude and humility for the care they receive, acknowledging that the caregiver (dentist or doctor) is offering their expertise and energy.

Patience and Perseverance: Healing, whether through dental care or other medical treatment, requires time and perseverance. Patients must practice patience, just as Arjuna is encouraged in the Gita to perform his duty with steadiness, no matter how difficult the path.

Patients practicing Karma Yoga should focus on the healing journey, not the immediate gratification of feeling better right away, but on the consistent effort of following.

Maintaining Faith and Positivity: One of the key teachings of Karma Yoga is maintaining faith and positivity throughout the journey, even when facing challenges. A patient's duty is to keep their mind uplifted, knowing that a positive outlook supports healing. This doesn't mean denying difficult emotions, but rather choosing to focus on hope and resilience. Patients must engage in their healing process with devotion—doing what is required, not out of fear or

Practical applications for patients:

Follow Medical Advice Without Attachment: Patients should stick to their treatment plan without overthinking the outcome, trusting that each step is getting them closer to health.

Reduce Mental Suffering by Letting Go: Rather than focusing on the potential agony of a dental surgery or anticipating future difficulties, patients can practice mindfulness, staying in the moment and letting the body to heal naturally.

Participate Actively: Karma Yoga promotes self-responsibility, which implies that patients actively participate in their rehabilitation by adhering to their health routines, such as regular oral hygiene, meditation, or following dietary recommendations.

Build Faith in the Process: Patients should have faith that the therapy, when carried out with the proper attitude and care, will result in healing, trusting both the practitioner and the healing process.

Rituals and affirmations for healthy teeth and gums:

The value of regular activities (rituals) and positive thinking (affirmations) in preserving oral health should not be overlooked.

The Bhagavad Gita emphasizes the importance of discipline and mindfulness in all aspects of life, and maintaining the health of your teeth and gums can be approached as a daily spiritual practice. Incorporating rituals and affirmations into oral hygiene not only improves physical health, but also aligns the mind and spirit with self-care and well-being. Establishing simple but meaningful rituals, such as brushing, flossing, and rinsing with care, can be viewed as an act of self-respect and gratitude for the body.

Verse 27, Chapter 9 of the Bhagvad Gita teaches that even routine tasks can become sacred when done with devotion. By approaching oral hygiene as a spiritual ritual, you honor your body and contribute to holistic wellness. Treat each step as a mindful act, and offer your practice to a higher purpose, ensuring you care for yourself as a reflection of divine creation.

Here are some examples of conscious oral care rituals:

Brushing with Intention: While brushing your teeth, picture removing not only physical plaque but also any bad thoughts or tension, which provides a deeper, spiritual connection to the cleansing process.

Tongue Scraping: Inspired by traditional Ayurvedic traditions, this can be a morning ritual to cleanse not only your mouth but also your communication channels, linking to the Gita's lessons on trut and self-expression.

Positive affirmations for healthy teeth and gums

The Bhagavad Gita emphasizes the power of the mind and thoughts in shaping reality, reminding us that inner harmony reflects outward. Affirmations are a powerful tool for aligning the mind with positive outcomes, so you can use them to reinforce your belief in health and vitality while caring for your teeth.

Bhagavad Gita: Chapter 6, Verse 6.

*bandhur ātmātmanas tasya yenātmaivātmanā jitaḥ
anātmanas tu śhatrutve vartetātmaiva śhatru-vat*

Translation: For one who has conquered the mind, it is the finest of allies; for one who has not, it remains the worst enemy."

These teachings can be used to educate patients and readers that maintaining a good perspective about their health benefits both the body and spirit. Include affirmations such as:

- "My teeth and gums are strong, healthy, and vibrant."
- "Every day, my oral health improves as I take care of my body and mind."
- "I nourish my body with love and care, and it reflects in my bright, healthy smile."

Patients can strengthen their mental commitment to health by repeating these affirmations on a regular basis, aligning their bodies with the spirit of healing and well-being.

Aligning Oral Health and Spiritual Growth

Brushing your teeth and saying affirmations every day aren't just for physical maintenance; they're also an opportunity to connect with your inner self, honor your body, and practice self-love. Taking conscious care of your teeth and gums embodies the discipline taught in the Bhagavad Gita and cultivates a holistic approach to health, where the mind, body, and spirit are all in sync.

The teachings of the Bhagavad Gita reveal that true wellness is not limited to physical appearance or health alone; it is a state of harmony between mind, body, and soul, which we cultivate step by step by approaching every aspect of our existence with awareness, discipline, and respect. Your teeth and gums are integral to this journey.

A New Perspective on Oral Health

As the Bhagvad Gita teaches us to see beyond the surface of things, we must also recognize that caring for our oral health is a sacred duty—a selfless act performed without attachment to the outcome, but with the deep understanding that every action contributes to our greater well-being. The Bhagavad Gita teaches us that the mind and body are interconnected, and that each of our actions creates ripples throughout our being. Neglecting oral health, or any aspect of our body, is a missed opportunity for growth and healing. By consciously caring for your teeth and gums, you embark on a journey of self-discovery.

A Call to Action: Mind, Body, and Spirit in Harmony

Every small act of self-care becomes part of a larger spiritual practice that nourishes not only your physical self but also your mental and emotional well-being. When you embrace this understanding, you activate the full potential of your life force and allow it to flow through you unhindered.

Key takeaways:

- Combining the wisdom of the Bhagavad Gita with practical spiritual practices can improve both the dentist's and patients' experiences.

- According to the Bhagvad Gita, Karma Yoga, or selfless action, is doing one's duty with attention and without attachment to the outcome, which can transform mundane chores into spiritual disciplines.

Conclusion

The Mouth is a Sacred Portal to Wholeness

As we near the end of this transformative journey through the hidden wisdom of oral health, it's critical to remember that your mouth is more than just a physical structure; it's a sacred portal that connects your mind, body, and spirit. Every tooth, breath, and word spoken reflects your inner world and the overall health of your being.

I urge you to embrace the practices and insights shared in this book, allowing you to take the first step towards integrating your dental wellness with your spiritual growth. You will learn that your smile is not only a reflection of happiness, but also a symbol of your soul's energy. Your teeth are not just tools for eating, but markers of your personal power and emotional history.

The rituals, practices, and perspectives presented here are more than just tools for maintaining dental hygiene; they are keys to unlocking a deeper understanding of yourself and your place in the universe. By caring for your oral health with mindfulness, reverence, and awareness, you are not only ensuring a healthy smile but also nurturing your spiritual essence.

As you continue on your path, keep in mind that true wellness is holistic. It's about balancing every aspect of your being—your thoughts, emotions, and physical health—with the divine energy that flows through you. Your mouth is the intersection of your inner and outer worlds, the physical and spiritual realms.

Let your journey not end here, but rather begin a lifelong practice of dental mindfulness, where every brushing, meal, and word is infused with intention and spiritual awareness. Accept the knowledge that by caring for your mouth, you are caring for your entire self—mind, body, and spirit. In the end, your mouth is a gateway not only to communication, but also to communion with the universe.

As you walk this route, may you smile with your heart as well as your mouth, knowing that your oral health reflects your soul's journey toward completeness and harmony.